UNORTHODOX FREUD

Permission to reprint the following material is gratefully acknowledged: Approximately 1,370 words from *My Analysis with Freud: Reminiscences* by Abram Kardiner. Copyright ©1977 by A. Kardiner. Reprinted by permission of Mrs. Ethel Diana Kardiner. Approximately 2,400 words from *Correspondence with Bryher MacPherson* by H. D. (Hilda Doolittle). Published by permission of the Beinecke Rare Book and Manuscript Library, Yale University. Approximately 1,100 words from *Tribute to Freud* by H. D. (Hilda Doolittle). Copyright ©1974 by Norma Haemes Pearson. Reprinted by permission of New Directions Publishing Corp. Approximately 2,860 words from *Fragments of an Analysis with Freud* by Joseph Wortis (reprinted in 1994 as *My Analysis with Freud*). Reprinted by permission of Jason Aronson, Inc. Approximately 945 words from *An American Psychiatrist in Vienna, 1935–1937, and His Sigmund Freud* by John M. Dorsey. Reprinted by permission of Edward C. Dorsey. Approximately 258 lines from *Diary of My Analysis with Sigmund Freud* by Smiley Blanton. Copyright ©1971 by Margaret Gray Blanton. Used by permission of Dutton Signet, a division of Penguin Books USA Inc. Approximately 135 lines from *The Standard Edition of the Complete Psychological Works of Sigmund Freud.* Reprinted by permission of Sigmund Freud Copyrights. Selected quotes from *The Collected Papers* (Vol. 2) by Sigmund Freud. Authorized translation under the supervision of Joan Riviere. Published by Basic Books, Inc., by arrangement with The Hogarth Press, Ltd., and the Institute of Psycho-Analysis, London. Reprinted by permission of BasicBooks, a division of HarperCollins Publishers, Inc.

UNORTHODOX FREUD
The View from the Couch

BEATE LOHSER, Ph.D.
PETER M. NEWTON, Ph.D.

THE GUILFORD PRESS
New York   London

©1996 The Guilford Press
A Division of Guilford Publications, Inc.
72 Spring Street, New York, NY 10012

Printed in the United States of America

This book is printed on acid-free paper.

Last digit is print number: 9 8 7 6 5 4 3 2 1

Library of Congress Cataloging-in-Publication Data available from
the Publisher.

ISBN 1-57230-128-7

Für Julian, Amelia, und Chelsea

[D]ie Antwort auf technische Fragen ist in der Psychoanalyse niemals selbstverständlich. Wenn es vielleicht mehr als nur einen guten Weg gibt, so gibt es doch sehr viele schlechte, und eine Vergleichung verschiedener Techniken kann nur aufklärend wirken, auch wenn sie nicht zur Entscheidung für eine bestimmte Methode führen sollte.

> —SIGMUND FREUD, "Die Handhabung der Traumdeutung in der Psychoanalyse" (1911, S. 151)

[T]he answer to questions of technique in analysis is never a matter of course. Although there may perhaps be more than one good road to follow, still there are very many bad ones, and a comparison of the various methods cannot fail to be illuminating, even if it should not lead to a decision in favour of any particular one.

> —SIGMUND FREUD, "The Handling of Dream-Interpretation in Psycho-Analysis" (1911, p. 91)

Acknowledgments

WE want to thank Maurice Marcus for reading early drafts of our book. His enthusiasm and thoughtful criticisms were essential in moving this project forward and helped identify some important problems. We are grateful as well to our editor, Kitty Moore, for seeing in the original manuscript something worth pursuing and for giving us the opportunity to do just that. Her suggestions for revisions were helpful in clarifying the direction and boundaries of our book. The Wright Institute helped in several ways, in particular by providing money for a research assistant, Pamela Simi. Ms. Simi diligently and expeditiously handled drafts and alerted us to the numerous small and big mistakes that kept appearing. At The Guilford Press, Judith Grauman distinguished herself once again by her extraordinarily competent production management, and Toby Troffkin was the very able copyeditor. Finally, our families and friends offered encouragement and emotional as well as practical support; Gene Riddle, in particular, generously lent to the preparation of the manuscript his computer expertise, which made that aspect of the work so much more tolerable.

Contents

UNORTHODOX FREUD

Introduction

IT may not seem possible to the psychoanalytic reader that another book on Freud's technique could offer anything new. After all, psychoanalysts and others have devoted considerable attention to the subject over the past several decades. Do we not know everything we need to know about how Freud treated his patients? In our opinion, the answer is "no." To the contrary, we find that the contemporary ideal of mainstream analytic treatment, which is called classical and attributed to Freud, is actually a post-World War II invention. This ideal centrally features abstinence, incognito, and neutrality and functions as a fixed reference point for adherence and deviation, both within the mainstream and beyond. While many mainstream psychoanalysts, perhaps especially among the most experienced, do not practice according to this ideal, it nonetheless operates not only as a powerful norm for students, the less experienced, and the less original, but also as inspiration for rebels.

In both current psychoanalytic literature and discourse, we encounter different versions of how Freud supposedly practiced psychoanalysis, simplifications that, like those our patients (not to mention ourselves!) proffer about their childhoods, stand badly in need of reanalysis. As a clinician, Freud has alternately been characterized as rigid and aloof, as overinvolved to the point of being unanalytic, or as having no technique at all. Of these depictions, the one that has prevailed has also become our foremost cliché of the "classical" analyst: "Freudian" in contemporary usage is widely assumed to mean detached, unresponsive, and cold.

In the discussion of Freud's clinical technique, the voices of his patients have not been fully heard. We hope with this book to offer a clearer understanding of how Freud actually did analysis by letting his

1

patients tell us themselves. Toward that end we present full narrative accounts and discussion of the five existing book-length reports by patients who were in analysis with Freud between 1921 and 1938. We analyze these treatments from a systems perspective in order to elucidate their structural principles. A secondary aim of this book is to contrast Freud's behavior with the position on technique he presented in his theoretical papers. A third is to look afresh at the value of Freud's legacy to us as contemporary clinicians.

Our knowledge of Freud's technique derives largely from two sources: his papers on treatment method and his published case histories. The fact that some discrepancy exists between the two was known to Freud and his followers during his lifetime and accepted as a matter of course. After Freud's death, however, the extent of these differences became exaggerated, creating an artificial split between his theory of technique and his work in practice. Moreover, while his theory of technique became the basis of the modern psychoanalytic ideal—eventuating in the stereotype of the Freudian analyst described above—Freud's standing as a therapist was diminished.

How can we understand the development that led to this split? A contributing factor at the methodological level is the fundamental incongruence between theory and application, which had made Freud leery of writing about technique to begin with. Furthermore, Freud expressed contradictory ideas about technique, which made his position on the subject vulnerable to the kind of polarization that was to occur later. Separating ideal from actual technique was likely motivated as well by political considerations and the desire to present a more acceptable version of the controversial new method to a potentially hostile audience. However, it appears that it was not until after the center of psychoanalytic thought and activity shifted to the United States following World War II that the gap broadened decisively. We will focus our analysis on this last point.

Lipton (1977), in his comparison of Freud's treatment of the Rat Man with modern technique, pointed out that during the 1950s modern technique had come to differ in crucial ways from Freud's—by separating the personal from the transference relationships, by emphasizing technique as a focus per se, and by postulating an ideal technique. For a variety of reasons, the distinction between Freud's practices and this new evolving theory of technique tended to get lost, and contradictions were resolved in favor of Freud's (presumed) theory, which was thought to more accurately reflect his views. The central tenets of the modern ideal were derived from Freud's seminal papers on technique, published between 1911 and 1915: The famous metaphors of the analyst as surgeon and as reflecting mirror, for example, trace back to these writings. However, only certain theoretical statements by Freud were selected for enshrinement as ideal; others were de-emphasized, and some were ignored entirely. Nonetheless, the new model of technique was retrospectively attributed to Freud and termed "classical." As we shall show, this ideal of classical technique, which continues to exert its influence over contemporary analytic clinicians, was a reinterpretation (sometimes a mistranslation) of Freud's ideas, not merely a restatement or summary of them.

Strachey's translation of Freud's German into the English *Standard Edition* hardened the authority in Freud's writings. Strachey set out, as he acknowledged, to render Freud into standard scientific English. As a result, whereas Freud used language poetically to suggest elusive psychological meanings, availing himself of the peculiar, rich, and (for foreign speakers) vexing variousness of German—in which multiple prefixes can be added or subtracted from the same verb to change its meaning—Strachey looked for a single English word to serve for every case. In other instances—and these have had, as we shall show, a very problematic and distorting effect upon our understanding of Freud's theory of technique— Freud's informality has been quite roughly forced into Edwardian attire. An appreciation of the particular effects of Strachey's strategy for translating Freud's German helps to restore the original element of relaxation and play in Freud's technical advice (see Ornston, 1992).

Accounts of Freud's actual clinical behavior have not received the same attention as his theoretical papers. Among the few such studies are those by Cremerius (1981) and Momigliano (1987). Cremerius's study includes clinical data from a variety of different sources—beginning with Freud's analysis of the Wolf Man in 1910 up to that of Smiley Blanton in 1938—and focuses especially on treatments reported by Freud's patients themselves. Cremerius presents his findings according to a priori categories such as the therapeutic climate, handling of the transference and resistance, interpretation, symbolic gratification, and so forth. The methodological problem of proceeding in this way (here and elsewhere) concerns the relevance of the categories. What if the most important patterns in the data do not fit them? Further, Cremerius presents anecdotal data in these categories without providing the treatment context for the particular examples. His main conclusion is that Freud's procedure was not very systematic, that is, that it was spontaneous, lively, and "artistic" rather than scientific.[1] It is to these aspects that Cremerius attributes the great variety of interventions and behaviors he found in the patients' reports.

Cremerius focuses his discussion on the "enormous" discrepancy he perceives between Freud's writings on procedure and the technique he practiced.[2] He believes that Freud presented a set of standards to the public and the medical establishment, namely, a scientific one, that he himself did not adhere to. The reasons for this, Cremerius suggests, can be attributed to the fact that Freud thought strict guidelines were necessary for those analysts who lacked the strength of character required to do responsible analytic work and to the fact that Freud wanted to protect psychoanalysis from the criticisms that its methods were unscientific and its practitioners simply human, that is, fallible, just like their patients. Although Cremerius's study is broad in scope and touches on a number of interesting points, the clinical data ultimately fail to transcend a level of anecdotal descriptiveness.

Momigliano's 1987 paper is similar to Cremerius's. She also analyzes reports by patients who were treated by Freud. Her primary interest is the clinical setting, and she discusses the process of acceptance for analysis, extra-analytic relations, the beginning phase, the sessions themselves, and termination. After presenting a number of interesting anecdotes, Momigliano concludes, as we have, that Freud did not behave like a mirror and that he spoke freely on various subjects. She notes a difference between, on the one hand, a level of ordinary communication between Freud and his patients that was not interpreted with respect to its transference implications and, on the other hand, a level of communication, involving dream material and spontaneous associations, that led to interpretations of the here-and-now relationship. She then raises a number of questions: Was Freud concerned about his countertransference getting in the way of the treatment? Did he keep real and transference relationships too separate from each other? Was he more interested in the original relationship than in the current transference? Instead of venturing to answer any of these questions, which she inexplicably finds "embarrassing," Momigliano writes shyly:

> Having reached this point, I realize, of course, that in order to conclude this paper fittingly I ought now to engage in a serious discussion of these matters, if possible attempting to formulate some intelligent hypotheses which might at least provide some interpretive suggestions and some replies to these embarrassing questions. . . . I must, however, admit that this does not interest me at all at this juncture.[3]

She adds that she wanted only to convey her fascination with the material itself—the atmosphere, the history, the patients' adventures with psychoanalysis and Freud. While Momigliano did this very well, the questions she posed need answers.

The majority of studies that examine Freud's clinical behavior isolate aspects of treatment and compare his interventions to contemporary standards, which do not always coincide with Freud's own. It is not surprising that most such studies conclude that Freud used a technique that differs from the current ideal. Unfortunately, rather than make an effort to understand exactly what Freud was trying to do and to examine specific interventions within this context, many researchers simply dismiss his clinical behavior as unorthodox. Most recently, Steven Ellman (1991) has claimed that Freud never mastered working with the transference, never fully left the pathogenic memory theory, and neither internalized his technique nor understood the full implications of his own thoughts.[4] He has also reissued the criticism that Freud was not a good clinician because he did not heed his own advice that analysts should be analyzed themselves.

In addition to doctrinal biases, the few studies of Freud's practice have suffered from inadequate data. Typically, such studies examine Freud's own case histories, such as those of Dora, the Rat Man, and the Wolf Man. The problem is that Freud wrote these cases to illustrate psychoanalytic conceptions of the mind and its aberrations, not to demonstrate his therapeutic method. They give us only condensed, composite examples of his technique. These pseudo examples lend themselves to the formation of theoretical stereotypes and cocktail party critiques of Freud's technical excesses. They are not, however, extensive enough to allow one to discover the order, stability, and reliable patterning that we have found Freud gave to his treatments. Though Thompson (1994) has recently come to views similar to the ones we published earlier (Lohser, 1988) about Freud's informality and personal engagement with his patients, his work, too, focuses upon the same limited case data. Longer narratives are required to present a rounded view of Freud's clinical work and to show, if they were different from our own, what his aims and means might have been.

In an effort to dismantle the stereotypes and resolve the contradictions, we present comprehensive narrative accounts and discussion of the only existing full-length reports written by analysands of Freud. These self-reports were produced by the following individuals: Abram Kardiner, analyzed in 1921–1922, a young American psychiatrist who would become an eminent social psychoanalyst; the famous American Imagist poet Hilda Doolittle (whose nom de plume was H.D.), analyzed in 1933 and 1934; Joseph Wortis, analyzed in 1934, who, like Kardiner, was a young American psychiatrist but one who would travel a very different path, introducing electroconvulsive shock therapy to the United States; and two other, lesser-known, American psychiatrists, both enthusiastic Christians—John Dorsey, whom Freud analyzed in 1935 and 1936, and Smiley Blanton, whom Freud analyzed in 1929 and 1930 and then on three separate occasions for brief periods during the 1930s, finally terminating in 1938.

These cases have never been studied together and rarely separately. This remarkable gap in the literature on Freud can only be explained by the relative lack of interest in his clinical, as opposed to his theoretical, work, as mentioned earlier. We think that these cases, especially presented together, are essential to our understanding of how Freud practiced psychoanalysis. All of the authors except H.D. present factual, chronological accounts of their treatments; we fashioned them into comprehensive narratives. H.D.'s story, however, cloudy, atemporal, and poetic, required more "treatment" on our part; we ordered the material in her *Tribute to Freud* to read coherently and fleshed it out with many passages from her fascinating, and still unpublished, correspondence with Bryher MacPherson.

Encumbered neither by the theoretical biases of Freud nor by those of his later commentators, these five accounts give us an intimate view of Freud at work. Most importantly, they are sufficiently extensive to permit us to identify the organizational principles that appear to have underlain Freud's behavior. We believe they constitute the best record available of what Freud actually did in treatment. Using these particular accounts as our primary data, however, also raises several concerns.

First, they are reminiscences, biographies, and pieces of literature rather than scientific treatises. Can these subjective portraits of Freud at work be trusted to have much objective value? We can only guess at the many reasons—some of them no doubt admirable and others more self-serving—that motivated these authors to write about their experiences with Freud and remember him in the particular ways they did. Moreover, although four of the reports are based on diaries and journal entries made at the time, Kardiner's was reproduced from memory years after the analysis had ended, making distortions of the original events seem inevitable. And finally, due to the nature of psychoanalytic work, one would expect each treatment to have its own particular character, varying according to diagnosis, personality style, and dynamics generated between patient and analyst. Can the picture of Freud that emerges from these accounts transcend their subjectivity and allow for valid generalizations concerning his technique? Cremerius (1981) answered this question in a convincing manner. He compared these patients' descriptions of Freud's technique with Freud's own accounts of his technique with the Rat Man—which he wrote as the case was actually proceeding—and the Wolf Man. Cremerius found that there were no significant differences between Freud's account and those of the patients. We came to the same conclusion after comparing Freud's case studies—and other more anecdotal accounts, such as those that appear in Ruitenbeek (1973)—with our five cases.

Second, the majority of the cases under review here were training analyses. Though psychoanalytic training was much less formal in Freud's time than it is today, can generalizations be made from these treatments to personal analyses? When Wortis asked Freud whether a didactic analysis differed from an ordinary analysis in any important respect, Freud answered:

> Not essentially . . . only insofar as the material and progress of the analysis is different. With a neurotic patient the analysis must follow the fluctuations of symptoms and *Widerstand* [resistance] and adapts itself to the state of the patient at any given time. With a healthy student, these fluctuations don't always occur unless he is neurotic to start with or becomes neurotic during the analysis.[5]

If there were no essential differences between a training and a personal analysis, why did Freud prefer students over neurotic patients after World War I? It appears that the reasons for his preference were that didactic analyses tended to be shorter and that he wanted to spread his influence. Perhaps, too, working with apprentice analysts permitted Freud the greater measure of collaboration he so enjoyed. As noted, Cremerius did not find a significant difference between Freud's treatments of the Rat Man and the Wolf Man, who were very neurotic, and those of his students, and neither have we.

Third, there is a question as to whether our cases are representative of Freud's final technique. His technique is generally believed to have been definitive by 1909 at the very latest; it probably had become so a few years earlier, when he added the 1905 postscript to the *Fragment of an Analysis of a Case of Hysteria* (1905). The five analyses presented here span a nearly 20-year period of Freud's life, from age 65 to 82, shortly before his death. The study thus provides a view of Freud's late, and by then certainly final, technique. Could his method in his later life perhaps be considered postfinal, reflecting the gay, devil-may-care disinhibition of growing senility and differing significantly from, for instance, the way he practiced psychoanalysis at age 53 with the Rat Man? We think the answer again is no; as noted, comparisons with the Rat Man (and earlier cases) show consistency in his technique over the entire second half of his life.

If we can take these cases as truly illustrative, how does one go about studying them? We began our work by asking not whether Freud was being analytic or not but, rather, by asking, What does it appear that Freud was trying to do, and how was he going about it? Thus, in studying the entire set of extant accounts, we asked ourselves not whether Freud was interpreting transference, being neutral, and maintaining the "frame" but, rather, How did Freud organize his work? Put more formally, in the language of the theory of open systems, which originated at the Tavistock Centre in London (Rice, 1963; Miller & Rice, 1967; see also Newton & Levinson, 1973; Eagle & Newton, 1981) we asked, What is the primary task of the treatment systems Freud created, and what sort of structure did he use to achieve it? The primary task is the end toward which the work is aimed and provides a rational basis for evaluating the efficacy of treatment structure.

As Miller and Rice wrote in *Systems of Organization* (1967), "organization is the means through which the enterprise secures the performance of its tasks."[6] We find this simple, flat, colorless statement to be one of the most arresting in all of social science. Consider the schools, institutes, clinics, hospitals, and government agencies in which we work and the haphazard, impulsive, mindless, even panicky way in which tasks get identified and defined, structure created, ignored, and changed; then consider the great importance of the goals being so irrationally pursued. In our field, the goal is nothing less than the health and well-being of patients and the knowledge and skill of the clinicians who treat them.

Analytic clinicians typically do not like systems language. Neither do we ordinarily like considerations that seem social rather than psychological, for these seem impersonal, even bureaucratic. Systems language has been overused over the past several decades and is, in any event, graceless. We would make no recourse to it were not the consequences of ignorance in matters concerning organizational and psychotherapeutic task and structure so dire and the necessity for clarity about them so urgent. Fritz Redlich, former dean of the Yale Medical School, who was both a psychoanalyst and a serious student of organizational life, used to insist that a determinant of treatment outcome in surgery equal in importance to patient pathology and surgical procedure is the state of intergroup relations between doctors and nurses on the ward. He was not joking; he meant it.

Any system, even one as small as the psychoanalytic dyad, that endures beyond a few meetings develops an external boundary and an internal structure. Clinicians can form the boundary and create the structure consciously with an eye on the task they are trying to achieve and can invite the patient's understanding and responsible collaboration, or they can allow the structure to accrue by the enactment of their identification with their own supervisors and analyst, by non-task-relevant personal preferences, or by precedent-forming accidents and to operate invisibly. The treatment enterprise will become structured one way or another—with fateful consequences for task performance.

In Chapter 1 we discuss Freud's theoretical position on technique, noting elements that have since been overemphasized and others that have been ignored. It is our view that even in his theoretical statements Freud was much less rigid regarding matters of technique than is usually depicted. Thus, the flexibility found in his actual treatment behavior is much more in keeping with his published prescriptions and proscriptions than is generally believed. While certain of his more authoritative statements concerning transference and resistance analysis, abstinence, and analytic incognito have come to represent the cornerstones of psychoanalytic technique, other recommendations, such as the importance of flexibility, tact, spontaneity, and openness, have been neglected in discussions of both his theoretical papers and his actual therapeutic style. In other words, the tension that existed in Freud's work between the poles of calculated restraint and spontaneous engagement has been lost.

In Chapters 2, 3, 4, 5, and 6 we present chronological narrative accounts of the treatments of Kardiner, H.D., Wortis, Dorsey, and Blanton, accounts derived from their own books and correspondences recounting their analyses. We shall see in each case that Freud allowed a unique relationship with his analysand to evolve naturally and that he participated in it, even as his task and method remained essentially the same. These relationships ranged widely in emotional tone. With Kardiner, Freud was both encouraging and uncompromising; with H.D., he was fascinated and passionately engaged; with Wortis, he was frustrated, argumentative, and critical; with Dorsey, he seemed generally friendly, if at times perhaps bored or even mildly exasperated; with Blanton, Freud remained sympathetic and generous even as Blanton evidenced a rivalrous transference.

We shall watch these patients struggling, in varying measure, to maintain a conscious idealization of their renowned analyst and to keep an unconscious competitive devaluation covered over. We shall also see them fighting to maintain the appearance and conviction of gratitude, despite their resentment at having made themselves so small by their idealization of Freud, and to suppress the many evidences of Freud's being merely human. In the case of Blanton and H.D. (and more ambiguously so for Kardiner and Dorsey), it appears that the patient really did like Freud but felt it necessary to keep the affectionate feelings unadulterated. In the case of the four psychiatrists, each had also to hide the wish to exploit and plunder Freud for his own career (to "make capital" out of the famous seer, as Blanton put it); toward each younger analysand Freud evidences an underlying grandpaternalism that issues naturally from his generational position.

In Chapter 7 we integrate our observations from the five cases into a coherent picture of how Freud practiced psychoanalysis. Our first aim in this analysis is to identify empirical patterns in the clinical data, but we will refer to Freud's theoretical papers to highlight continuities and departures.

In Chapter 8 we present a historical sketch of the evolution of psychoanalytic technique from Freud's to the "basic model technique," which was introduced by Eissler in the 1950s and which continues to constitute a *neo*-orthodoxy that is mistakenly considered to be traditional. An understanding of the transmogrification of Freud's suggestions about technique into a neo-orthodox ideal of asepsis has more to offer than a correction of the historical record. This ideal continues to operate as a norm to be conformed to or deviated from by analytic practitioners both within the mainstream and outside of it. Consequently, much of the debate between "classical" and "newer" approaches to psychoanalysis proceeds, we believe, from a fundamentally mistaken premise of what constitutes classical psychoanalysis. In fact, the term "classical" has become such a confusing one that Wallerstein (1995) may be right in suggesting that it has outlived its usefulness for psychoanalysis. In Chapter 9 we offer a summary of our conclusions about the differences between Freud's approach to analytic treatment and the neo-orthodox ideal. We also point out some important advantages in Freud's therapeutic method. We believe strongly, with Lipton, that Freud's technique is important for current thinking, especially with respect to questions regarding neutrality, abstinence, and the analytic relationship. We also believe that Freud's way of participating in the work of analysis has implications not only for our professional development as clinicians but also for our personal development as adults.

Over the years, there have been recurrent debates within mainstream psychoanalysis and beyond concerning the necessity of neutrality and abstinence. To us, what is at stake here is the adult development of the clinician and the extent to which a proper place exists for its expression in the work or treatment. Momigliano (1987) asked the seemingly preposterous question, Was Freud a Freudian? We shall attempt to make clearer what it means to be Freudian and to answer a second question as well: Shouldn't we be? Along the way, we shall make the surprising discovery that Freud's relationships to his patients appear to have been less tilted than our own and characterized by a greater degree of collaboration. How can this be? Was Freud not a paternalistic Victorian? Are we not postmodern egalitarians? We shall show the greater equality resulted from Freud's organizing his treatments differently.

Freud's Theory of Technique

IN the following pages we will summarize Freud's theoretical position on technique. Our purpose here is not to revisit the familiar discussion of his major concepts but to provide a brief account of his most important procedural guidelines and, particularly, to highlight ones that have been largely ignored, namely, those calling for flexibility and tact. We will see that Freud did not generally believe that rules of technique could or should be rigidly applied; his were not meant to constitute an absolute or ideal of analytic behavior. There were exceptions, however, points where Freud was speaking with *ex cathedra* authority. He *was* adamant about the importance of free association and sexual abstinence, and he considered the analysis of the transference and the handling of resistances absolute treatment prerequisites—although, as we shall see, he did not place transference analysis at the center of treatment, as is often the case today, and working with the resistance meant something quite different to Freud than resistance analysis means to contemporary clinicians. What we wish to emphasize is that although the voice of authority is counterbalanced by a more tentative one, it is mainly the voice of dogma that has carried over the years.

During a half century of clinical work and in some 300 scientific publications, Freud wrote relatively little on the subject of technique. Between 1895 and 1937, he dedicated some 20 papers—not counting the case studies whose primary purpose was to prove the validity of scientific hypotheses, not to demonstrate his therapeutic method—to the question of what principles should guide the analyst in conducting a psychoanalytic treatment. Of these, only a handful are original and explicit in technical instruction. The remainder are either prepsychoanalytic in nature or are general overviews and summaries of previously stated ideas, such as the *Introductory Lectures on Psycho-Analysis* (1916–1917).

FREUD'S *RATSCHLÄGE*

Of particular importance among these writings is a collection of six papers, published between 1911 and 1915, that represents Freud's only attempt at a systematic outline of his procedure. He had originally planned to write a small handbook to be called "Allgemeine Technik der Psychoanalyse" (A General Account of the Psychoanalytic Technique), but after several postponements published his ideas instead in this series of six articles.[1] It is from these papers that principles guiding psychoanalytic treatment have been generalized, and they can be said to form the foundation of classical psychoanalytic technique.

It appears from the scarcity of his writings on technique that Freud may have been reluctant to formally articulate his views on psychoanalytic method, and there is other evidence to support this notion. Uncharacteristically, Freud had procrastinated with the formulation and publication of the originally planned handbook (Mitscherlich, Richards, & Strachey, 1982). In his biography of Freud, Jones (1955) pointed out that the idea of a handbook giving a fuller account of the psychoanalytic method first came up during the Salzburg Congress in 1908, a conference that gave Freud a clearer idea of the extent to which interest in psychoanalytic treatment was growing. He began the project six months later, but after a number of delays he abandoned the idea of a textbook and instead decided to write a group of essays.[2] It was another 18 months before the first of the six papers, which Freud himself regarded as forming a series,[3] was published in December 1911; the last one appeared in January 1915. Over the next 25 years of energetic psychoanalytic writing, he would offer only two more original pieces on method (Freud, 1937a, 1940a).

What were the reasons for Freud's reticence to give a detailed outline of his technique? Several problems—some intrinsic to the subject, others extrinsic—can be identified. Above all, Freud felt (and he emphasized this repeatedly) that a systematic and exhaustive account of his procedure was not possible. He worried about giving his followers guidelines that would necessarily be imprecise and incomplete, but he also did not want his patients to know too much about his method. Moreover, Freud did not relish the idea of potentially supplying his opponents with further ammunition against psychoanalysis (Mitscherlich et al., 1982). At the time he was first considering writing about technique, he was still greatly concerned about the reaction of the scientific community to his new treatment: How could he convince his fellow physicians to take his talking cure seriously if details about its method revealed what might appear as rather vague and unscientific proceedings? Freud had expressed his concern about this several years before the technique papers were published:

> To many physicians, even to-day, psychotherapy seems to be the offspring of modern mysticism and, compared with our physico-chemical specifics which are applied on the basis of physiological knowledge, appears quite unscientific and unworthy of the attention of a serious investigator.[4]

Ellman (1991) has offered yet another plausible reason for Freud's hesitation about publishing technical papers: Freud's desire to leave open the possibility of future changes in psychoanalytic technique and to avoid committing himself to a prematurely finished version. It is most likely as a result of all these considerations that Freud at first intended to distribute the proposed handbook privately among the analysts in his small and trusted circle, a fact we know from Jones (1955).

In *Freud and His Followers*, Roazen (1975) agrees that Freud seemed hesitant to write on the subject of technique and suggests that he changed his mind only following dissension in the movement: "He had been reluctant to write about his special approach until his quarrels with Adler, Stekel, and Jung, when it seemed advisable to distinguish his own form of treatment from that of other psychotherapists."[5] Jones supports this view and adds that after the first two papers on technique were written in 1912—one on dream interpretation and the other on transference—"Freud's wish to give fuller instruction to those employing his methods was strengthened by the unhappy dissensions that had recently taken place, which he felt sure were largely due to the correct procedure not being adhered to."[6] He therefore decided to give an outline of general technical rules and principles in the last four essays, which resulted in the special subgroup of four among the six papers entitled "Recommendations to Physicians Practising Psycho-Analysis."

Most importantly, however, it was Freud's skepticism about the usefulness of establishing strict rules in the training of future analysts that restrained him. He believed that only general guidelines could be laid down and that their application had to be left to tact and experience, particularly in the form of a training analysis:

> It is not enough, therefore, for a physician to know a few of the findings of psycho-analysis; he must also have familiarized himself with its technique if he wishes his medical procedure to be guided by a psycho-

analytic point of view. This technique cannot yet be learnt from books, and it certainly cannot be discovered independently without great sacrifices of time, labour and success. Like other medical techniques, it is to be learnt from those who are already proficient in it.[7]

Freud emphasized repeatedly that academic or theoretical knowledge could not substitute for experience in learning the psychoanalytic method.

Fenichel, too, believed that the most decisive reason for the general scarcity of writings on psychoanalytic technique was that "the infinite multiplicity of situations arising in analysis does not permit the formulation of general rules about how the analyst should act in every situation, because each situation is essentially unique."[8] In a fitting analogy, Freud likened the analytic process to the game of chess, in which only opening moves and some typical ending constellations allow for systematic depiction. What goes on in between cannot be learned from books:

> The extraordinary diversity of the psychical constellations concerned, the plasticity of all mental processes and the wealth of determining factors oppose any mechanization of the technique; and they bring it about that a course of action that is as a rule justified may at times prove ineffective, whilst one that is usually mistaken may once in a while lead to the desired end.[9]

In the same paper Freud uses the German term *Spielregeln* (*Spiel* meaning "play" or "game" and *Regeln* meaning "rules"), or "rules to a game which acquire their importance from their relation to the general plan of the game,"[10] to suggest that flexibility and even playfulness are essential ingredients in the application of his technical suggestions. It should be noted in this context that Strachey's rendering of Freud's "Ratschläge für den Arzt bei der psychoanalytischen Behandlung" in the *Standard Edition* as "Recommendations to Physicians Practising Psycho-Analysis" is misleading. *Ratschläge* should have been translated as "pieces of advice" (*Rat* means "advice"; *Schläge* means, in this context, "bits, pieces"), not "recommendations." Pieces of advice are avuncular and friendly and not necessarily of the weight of professional judgment that is ignored at one's peril. It is true that Freud does occasionally make recommendations—as well as set down more binding rules—in the text of these articles, but if he had wanted to emphasize recommendations, he would have used the word for them—*Empfehlungen*.

Even though the more definitive and authoritative term "rule" (*Regel*) does appear in his technical writings, Freud applied it with consistency only to the fundamental rule of free association (i.e., *Grundregel*). Frequently, he offered advice and suggestions instead. He wrote, for example, "I think I am well-advised, however, to call these rules 'recommendations' [again, this should read "pieces of advice"] and not to claim any unconditional acceptance for them."[11]

In many instances Freud presented alternative choices to what might be considered standard procedure and merely warned the analyst who employs them to be prepared for the consequences. A case in point is a comment about the difficulties that can arise if the analyst accepts into treatment a person with whom he has social ties, such as a friend's wife or child. This can "have special disadvantageous consequences for which one must be prepared. . . . [The analyst] must be prepared for it to cost him that friendship, no matter what the outcome of the treatment may be: nevertheless he must make the sacrifice if he cannot find a trustworthy substitute."[12] We know that Freud made this particular kind of exception with his daughter Anna. Ellman (1991) has speculated that analyzing Anna might have seemed necessary to Freud because he did not trust anyone else with the task.

Freud pointed out that individual differences in the analyst's personality make the prescription of definitive rules for his conduct difficult as well. More than once he cautioned the reader that his technique had proven to be the only one compatible with his own personality: "I must however make it clear . . . that this technique is the only one suited to my individuality; I do not venture to deny that a physician quite differently constituted might find himself driven to adopt a different attitude to his patients and to the task before him."[13]

TAKT

Considering the strong emphasis Freud placed on flexibility in the application of his procedural guidelines, it is interesting to note, as Roazen pointed out, that many of his followers treated them as rigid rules. As early as 1928 Freud complained about this tendency in a letter to Ferenczi, who had just written a paper called "The Elasticity of Psycho-Analytic Technique." Freud applauded him for the excellent title and continued:

> The "Recommendations on Technique" I wrote long ago were essentially of a negative nature. I considered the most important thing was to emphasize what one should *not* do, and to point out the temptations in directions contrary to analysis. Almost everything positive that one *should* do I have left to "tact." . . . The result was that the docile analysts did not perceive the elasticity of the rules I had laid down, and submitted to them as if they were taboos. Sometime all that must be revised, without, it is true, doing away with the obligations I had mentioned.[14]

The German *Takt*, which in addition to the English meaning of "tact" also refers to timing in music, is used here to suggest the analyst's intuitive sense of what to do at any given time, rather than politeness. The narrower English connotation has contributed to the neglect of Freud's emphasis on intuition and flexibility in the interpretation of his papers. Thus, his reminder "Everything positive that one *should* do I have left to tact" has not been taken seriously enough. It is also true, however, that Freud did not attempt to define more formally his understanding of tact or intuition as a tool in analytic treatment; he thought of it as a special ability related to the analyst's personality and experience and, hence, a difficult quality to impart. In the letter to Ferenczi quoted above, Freud said about tact:

> All those who have no tact will see in what you write a justification for arbitrariness, i.e. subjectivity, i.e. the influence of their own un-mastered complexes. What we encounter in reality is a delicate balancing—for the most part on the preconscious level—of the various reactions we expect from our interventions. The issue depends above all on a quantitative estimate of the dynamic factors in the situation. One naturally cannot give rules for measuring this; the experience and the normality of the analyst have to form a decision. But with beginners one therefore has to rob the idea of "tact" of its mystical character.[15]

Freud attempted to do so by offering some rules and guidelines that adequate tact would make unnecessary. As early as 1910 he wrote: "Besides all this, one may sometimes make a wrong surmise, and one is never in a position to discover the whole truth. Psycho-analysis provides these definite technical rules to replace the indefinable 'medical tact' which is looked upon as some special gift."[16] Freud did not regard it as a special gift. Thus he told Kardiner, when the latter marveled at Freud's exceptional ability to interpret dreams, that it was not a special talent but, rather, the ready availability of his counterassociations. In his paper "The Elasticity of Psycho-Analytic Technique" Ferenczi (1928) offered another definition of tact: "But what is 'tact'? The answer is not very difficult. It is the capacity for empathy."[17]

TREATMENT ESSENTIALS

Between tact on the one hand and pieces of advice on the other, what were the obligations that Freud believed could not be dispensed with in psychoanalytic treatment? A review of his papers on technique from 1900 onward reveals that there were but a few. In the following pages we briefly summarize the most important rules Freud proposed to govern the analyst's conduct and general attitude.

Free Association, Resistance, Transference, and Abstinence

Above all, Freud insisted on the overriding importance of the fundamental rule, free association, and emphasized that the conditions of the treatment *must* ensure the patient's spontaneous verbal expression. He advised analysts to explain this rule to their patients in the first hour and to monitor their adherence to it. In "On Beginning the Treatment," Freud (1913a) suggested helping the patient understand the requirement of free association by telling him to act like a traveler on a train who, sitting at the window, describes everything he sees outside to fellow travelers who do not share his view. Freud considered free association to be central because it paves the way for uncovering resistances, unconscious conflicts, and repressed memories.

Throughout his technical papers, Freud emphasized the importance of working with the resistance. We use the phrase "working with the resistance" advisedly; in our reading of Freud, we did not come across a single instance in which he referred to "analyzing" the resistance. Freud spoke most commonly about "overcoming" resistance; he also used the terms "fighting," "tackling," "uncovering," and "doing away with" resistance, but he never referred to "analyzing" it as in modern usage. For example, in "Remembering, Repeating and Working-Through" Freud (1914a) said:

> [T]he resistance had become all the stronger, and the whole situation was more obscure than ever. The treatment seemed to make no headway. . . . The treatment was as a rule progressing most satisfactorily. The analyst had merely forgotten that giving the resistance a name could not result in its immediate cessation. One must allow the patient time to become more conversant with this resistance with which he has now become acquainted, to *work through* it, to overcome it, by continuing, in defiance of it, the analytic work according to the fundamental rule of analysis.[18]

Freud explained in his paper on "Wild Psycho-Analysis" (1910c) that presenting patients with revelations about their unconscious is not sufficient in the fight against resistance:

> If knowledge about the unconscious were as important for the patient as people inexperienced in psycho-analysis imagine, listening to lectures or reading books would be enough to cure him. Such measures, however, have as much influence on the symptoms of nervous illness as a distribution of menu-cards in a time of famine has upon hunger.[19]

Giving in to the temptation of guessing our patients' unconscious secrets from their associations, the procedure referred to as "wild," would contribute little, Freud is saying, to the working through of resistances. At worst, it might mean losing the patient. Freud knew about this danger from experience. He remarked in several places that his own impatience had cost him analysands, and we know from case material that interpreting deep material early continued to be a temptation Freud often could not resist.

However, as Gray (1994) points out in a paper on the "developmental lag" in the application of ego psychology to analytic technique, Freud vacillated throughout his writings between two positions regarding interpretation: On the one hand, analysts are to wait for their patients to get close to the discovery of unconscious material themselves before making an interpretation; on the other hand, telling patients before they themselves have gotten there can help establish "a 'record' or impression, in consciousness, of what is presumed to exist as a separate record in the repressed unconscious."[20] Gray calls this the "two-records" approach and points out that as late as 1937, in his paper "Constructions in Analysis," Freud defended the second strategy and wrote that the purpose of creating such an impression in the patient's consciousness was "so that it may work on him."[21]

Although there is a contradiction in his writings regarding the usefulness for the patient of conscious knowledge about the origins of his illness and the meaning of his symptoms, it is also true that more often than not Freud rejects taking "an intellectualist view of the situation."[22] He says in most places that interpretations usually will not help unless two conditions have been met: "First, the patient must, through preparation, himself have reached the neighbourhood of what he has repressed, and secondly, he must have formed a sufficient attachment (transference) to the physician for his emotional relationship to him to make a fresh flight impossible."[23]

In the transference patients repeat in their relationships with the analyst early unresolved conflicts with their parents; transference therefore constitutes an "intermediary region between illness and real life."[24] Freud considered the resolution of the transference one of the main goals of analytic treatment.[25] He writes:

> This struggle between the doctor and the patient, between intellect and instinctual life, between understanding and seeking to act, is played out almost exclusively in the phenomena of transference. It is on that field that the victory must be won—the victory whose expression is the permanent cure of the neurosis. . . . For when all is said and done, it is impossible to destroy anyone *in absentia* or *effigie*.[26]

The transference is usually ambivalent, as are children's relationships with their parents. In its positive form it manifests as affection for and the wish to please the analyst and gain his or her love; it motivates the patient to get well and is therefore a necessary condition for successful treatment. In its negative or eroticized forms, however, the transference becomes the source of the strongest resistance. It is at this point that the transference is interpreted: "*So long as the patient's communications and ideas run on without any obstruction, the theme of transference should be left untouched.* One must wait until the transference, which is the most delicate of all procedures, has become a resistance."[27] Freud did not say anywhere in his writings that the transference makes up the entirety of the relationship between patient and analyst. He did not address, however, except in passing, what was later called the "real relationship" (see Greenson, 1967).

One rule Freud is adamant about in his theoretical papers is that of abstinence from sexual contact with patients. Analysts should also abstain from being too gratifying with regard to their patients' attempts to seek relief from their neurotic condition; that is, they should refuse to satisfy demands that are intrinsic to the patient's conflict. However, Freud concedes that it is not possible to withhold from the patient every human gratification; the analyst will have to decide what those limits are in each individual case. Again, this is not presented as a rigid rule; much is left to the analyst's judgment and tact. The clinician must be sufficiently flexible to maintain a balance between frustration and gratification in terms of both the shifting tolerances of the patient and the enduring requirements of the task (see Newton, 1971).

A particular kind of attitude on the analyst's part is most conducive for the overall aim of treatment. Freud sums up the pertinent rules in the following words:

> They are all intended to create for the doctor a counterpart to the "fundamental rule of psycho-analysis" which is laid down for the patient. Just as the patient must relate everything that his self-observation can detect . . . so the doctor must put himself in a position to make use of everything he is told for the purposes of interpretation and of recognizing the concealed unconscious material without substituting a censorship of his own for the selection that the patient has foregone. To put this in a formula: he must turn his own unconscious like a receptive organ towards the transmitting unconscious of the patient. . . . [S]o the doctor's unconscious is able, from the derivatives of the unconscious which are communicated to him, to reconstruct that unconscious, which has determined the patient's free associations.[28]

This state of mind is also referred to as "evenly-suspended attention."[29] It decreases the strain of listening and ensures that the analyst will not focus selectively on the material: "In making the selection, if he follows his expectations he is in danger of never finding anything but what he already knows; and if he follows his inclinations he will certainly falsify what he may perceive."[30] To allow for this kind of unfocused attention, analysts must be aware of their countertransference reactions and the potential effect of these on the treatment. Freud advised that analysts undergo a didactic analysis not only to learn about technique firsthand but to work through their own conflicts and resistances, thus preventing "blind spots"[31] from interfering with their work. Interestingly, in 1912 Freud still thought that analyzing one's own dreams could in some cases be sufficient preparation for becoming an analyst. He felt this had been true in his own case, and although he expressed mixed opinions over the years about the adequacy of this sort of preparation, the possibility remained close to his heart (Masson, 1985; Freud, 1910a, 1937).

One of the first tasks of treatment is to attach the patient to the analyst, a development that is promoted by an analytic stance characterized by empathy, serious interest, and acceptance. This, together with instructions about free association and the removal of initial resistances, is sufficient to help patients express themselves more freely. Freud remarked in this context as well that interpretations should not be made before a good working alliance has been established, warning analysts that "these kinds of lightning diagnoses and 'express' treatments" will only intensify resistances or even lead to premature termination.[32]

Analysts are, moreover, to be honest (in the sense of lacking pretense) and direct about matters that are usually treated as taboos, like money and sex. The analyst must also be respectful of patients' individuality and help them realize their own potential rather than model them after his or her personal ideals. At times, however, the situation may require the analyst to function in the role of guide and educator.

Neutrality

In seeming contradiction to the kind and sympathetic attitude just described are several often quoted suggestions that were later summarized under the concept of "neutrality," a topic of central importance to modern psychoanalytic technique. Because of its importance, we will discuss this topic in detail at a later point. A short summary will suffice here. In his paper "Recommendations to Physicians Practising Psycho-Analysis," Freud (1912c) suggested that the analyst should be like a mirror and reflect back to the patient only what is shown to him or her; this is a warning about the consequences of too much personal disclosure on the part of the clinician as a means of overcoming the patient's resistances.

Another of Freud's treatment metaphors, that of the analyst as surgeon, later became influential in shaping the concept of the analytic attitude: Freud recommended that the analyst proceed with "emotional coldness" and put all his feelings aside, "even his human sympathy."[33] This is a reminder that at times analysts have to ignore their feelings of compassion and empathy. In other words, their kindness must ultimately be subordinated to the task of the analysis, which by its very nature involves suffering on the patient's part. Rather than constituting a prescription for an overall approach to treatment—a later interpretation of these passages in Freud's writings—his statements address particular procedural difficulties. At the same time, however, the choice of meta-phors suggests a retreat to the researcher-scientist stance in clinical situations in which the analyst is presented with particular emotional temptations. With this imagery, Freud added an objective, scientific dimension to his technical guidelines, which stands in contrast to the subjective and intuitive approach he generally suggested the analyst adopt. We will return to this problem later.

Dream Analysis

Another central treatment focus for Freud is the work with dreams. As is well known, his self-analysis featured the study of the associated moods and memories that accompanied his dreams. Indeed, as noted previously, his first answer to the question of how one becomes an analyst cited the study of one's own dreams.[34] Considering Freud's enduring passion for dreams, it is not surprising that the first of his papers on technique (1911a) is a discussion of the place and interpretation of dreams in psychoanalysis. In that paper he nonetheless points out that the work with dreams should not be assigned special status, but should follow the same guidelines as the rest of the treatment; in other words, dream interpretation should not be "pursued as an art for its own sake."[35] But again Freud concedes, "Occasionally, of course, one can at times act otherwise and allow a little free play to one's theoretical interest; but one should always be well aware of what one is doing."[36] Freud warns that dreams are often used for the purpose of resistance, which can manifest itself in the patient bringing in more dream material than can be handled in a given hour. Analysts should therefore be content, Freud suggests, with "the amount of inter-pretation which can be achieved in one session . . . and it is not to be regarded as a loss if the content of the dream is not fully discovered."[37]

The Analyst's Behavior

In his overall suggestions Freud was not very specific with respect to the analyst's actual behavior. In fact, he addressed himself to this point in only two of the technique papers. It seems that his interest was in creating a treatment situation that would be most conducive for achieving the goal of the analysis rather than in establishing rigid rules or standards of conduct for their own sake. This is an important point about Freud's orientation toward matters of procedure: In the end, the primary task (in the sense of ultimate goal or mission), the raison d'être of the treatment, determines the analyst's interventions. The analyst's behavior (within certain limits), in and of itself, is of only secondary significance. In modern discussions technique, such as analyzing the transference, is often unwittingly lifted from the status of a method to the level of a goal. This is an example of what Eagle and Newton (1981) have called "task displacement," an unconscious phenomenon common in human services enterprises, where the long-term or ultimate success of one's work is hard to measure. Freud was exceedingly task oriented, in his clinical work as well as in his research. What mattered to him most were results, not methods. Because of this basic orientation, Freud contented himself with outlining in his papers the contours of the analytic situation and the analyst's behavior; he filled in the spaces only with the understanding that tact and experience would ultimately shape the particular course of a given treatment.

Freud (1913a) makes a number of specific suggestions in "On Beginning the Treatment." None, however, is really binding, and much is left to the analyst's preference and tact. He suggests, for instance, an initial trial period of two weeks before accepting a patient for psychoanalysis. Himself in his 50s when he wrote this paper, Freud suggests that the patient should not be this old, lest he or she be too inflexible psychologically. He opines that the patient's being moderately educated is a help. Drawing upon his own 10-year experiment with pro bono treatment. Freud warns against seeing the patient for too little money. The financial recompense plays an important role in the transference and in the degree of the patient's suffering and sacrifice. Analysts who agree to a low fee need to be aware of possible deleterious consequences for the work. Freud suggests that analysts adopt the notion of renting out their time to patients, who will be responsible for payment even when they miss an appointment, and that when the nature and progress of a case warrant it, the number of visits per week can be reduced from the more usual six to three. However, it is generally advisable, he writes, to begin treatment with more frequent visits, and it might also be necessary occasionally to lengthen meetings beyond the usual 60-minute session, even to the extent of doubling the original amount of time. Freud recommends that the patient agree not to make significant life decisions while in treatment and not to study psychoanalytic theory.

Thus, in his technical advice Freud shifts back and forth between

two positions: He presents an overall treatment approach that is characterized by flexibility, tact, and individual preference, an approach in
which interventions arise from the context of the treatment situation,
which includes the analyst's and patient's personalities and clinical
requirements. On the other hand, he issues more absolute and authoritative directives with reference to free association, analysis of transference, abstinence, neutrality, and the uncovering and overcoming of
resistance.

This kind of duality is a reflection both of Freud's personality and of
the dialectical nature of psychoanalytic theory. With regard to the former,
Freud was a man of strong feelings who was guided in his work by
intuition. Indeed, he derived fundamental psychoanalytic insights from
the self-analysis occasioned by his own mid-life crisis (Newton, 1995).
In his approach to treatment he was intensely personal as well as impersonal, scientific, and authoritative. But while it is important to consider
what personal characteristics may have contributed to these apparent
contradictions in the theory, it would be reductionistic to leave it at
that.[38]

In Freud's view, psychoanalytic theory and its subject matter are
fundamentally dialectic. Consequently, such polarities are present in the
technique of treatment, placing it in between art and science, free
association and structure, subjectivity and objectivity, tact and rules,
personality and formality. Freud did not attempt to resolve these polarities. Both aspects are ineluctable in life, in persons, and therefore in his
theory, and decisions about particular behaviors or interventions must
come out of a particular context. Freud did not offer simple, one-dimen-
sional, clear-cut solutions but kept, even in his theory of technique, the
complexity of the analytic enterprise at the center. Herein lies one source
of the richness and durability of psychoanalytic theory in general and
therapeutic procedure in particular.

In the 1950s, the theory of technique in the United States lost some
of this richness and the polarity collapsed into a theory that emphasized
the rational, objective, impersonal, scientific, and rule-bound aspects of
the original. The banished pole of tact, empathy, intimacy, and spontaneity—"intersubjectivity" in its most recent garb—tended to split off
from mainstream psychoanalysis into separate schools. After immersing
ourselves in the clinical data and, in Chapter 7, deriving the principles
upon which Freud appears to have organized these treatments, we shall
consider in Chapter 8 some reasons why the theory of technique that still
functions as ideal in mainstream psychoanalysis became so imbalanced.

Freud's Analysis
of Abram Kardiner

ABRAM Kardiner was born in New York City on August 17, 1891, the son of Isaac and Mildred Kardiner. He was educated at the City College of New York and earned his M.D. degree from Cornell University in 1917. After his analysis with Freud was completed in 1922, Kardiner returned to New York, where he became one of the founders of the New York Psychoanalytic Society, the first training institute of its kind. In 1945, together with Drs. S. Rado, D. Levy, and G. Daniels, Kardiner cofounded the first psychoanalytic training school connected with a university medical school at Columbia. Here they refined their Adaptational Theory, which formed the basis of Kardiner's social psychoanalytic research of illiterate and modern societies. Kardiner emphasized the influence of culture on the development of the individual, and he created a unique method for studying the person within his or her social context. This method combined data from relevant institutional settings with data collected from personal biographies, dreams, and psychological tests. The results of this research are contained in his book *The Psychological Frontiers of Society* (1945) as well as in some of his other works. In 1962, *Science* magazine honored Kardiner for his "original and substantive contributions" to the field of social science. Kardiner married late in life, at 57, and had one daughter, Ellin. He died in 1981 at the age of 89. All of the following quotes are from Kardiner's book *My Analysis with Freud* (1977), unless otherwise noted. Kardiner was 30 at the time of the analysis; Freud was 65.

Freud focused in this treatment on the analysis of the Oedipus complex and unconscious homosexuality. Dream analysis was central in the unraveling of these dynamics, as was Kardiner's history; Freud did not address the here-and-now transference. He interpreted Kardiner's anger and defiance only genetically, which Kardiner later thought of as a failure that perpetuated his difficulty with self-assertion. Despite this and other criticisms, Kardiner thought that the analysis was a "brilliant perform-ance done with speed and accuracy."

* * *

Abram Kardiner began his analysis with Freud in the fall of 1921. He had contacted Freud in the beginning of the year to inquire about the possibility of working with him. Had it not been for H. W. Frink, his former training analyst, Kardiner would never have dared approach Freud; he was a novice in the field and saw no special reason why this famous man should be interested in him. Frink himself was at that time in analysis with Freud and told Kardiner that he, too, would benefit greatly from such an opportunity; he encouraged him to apply and promised to put in a good word on his behalf.[1] To Kardiner's surprise, he received this letter from Freud in late April 1921:

> I am glad to accept you for analysis especially since Dr. Frink has given so good an account of you. . . . Six months are a good term to achieve something both theoretically and personally. You are requested to be in Vienna on the first of October, as my hours will be given away shortly after my return from the vacation. . . . My fees are $10.00 an hour or about $250 monthly to be paid in effective notes, not in checks which I could only change for crowns.[2]

Freud had another request, namely, that the analysis be conducted in German if possible, but Kardiner was not sufficiently fluent in that language.[3] Kardiner was thrilled at the prospect of being analyzed by Freud himself. He had four months to make the necessary arrangements for his trip abroad; he saved what money he could, borrowed the rest, and was off to Europe in the late summer.

Kardiner arrived in Vienna at the end of September 1921. A small group of Freud's analysands were already gathered there. Five were from the United States, three were from England, and one was from Switzer-land; the majority were students.[4] One of them was Monroe Meyer, an American colleague who had started his treatment with Freud several months earlier. He helped Kardiner find accommodations and suggested that they meet Freud at the railway station upon his return from an extended summer vacation. On Sunday, September 29, 1921, Kardiner caught his first glimpse of Freud as he got off the train. At first he was disappointed: Freud was shorter than he had imagined, and his voice was hoarse. However, Kardiner was soon impressed with Freud's perfect

command of English and his air of authority. Freud was friendly, introduced the two Americans to his family and maid, and asked that they
meet him at his office the following day. This brief encounter left
Kardiner feeling that Freud was someone he could trust; he was also
immediately convinced that his affiliation with this famous man would
be helpful both personally and professionally.

THE FIRST CLINICAL ENCOUNTER

Analyst and patient met at the appointed time for a preliminary interview. Freud asked for biographical information, which Kardiner provided
in abbreviated form. On the subject of his training analysis with Frink,
the following conversation transpired:

> "And what did you get out of your analysis with Dr. Frink?" to which
> I replied, "Nothing," and went on with my story. At the end of forty
> minutes, he said, "I think you are a very interesting personality to work
> with, but you made one statement which I would like to correct. You
> said you got nothing out of your analysis with Frink. You are wrong.
> You did get something out of it." "What did I get?" To which Freud
> replied laconically, "A little neurosis."[5]

When the session was almost over, Freud announced that there was a
problem: He was in the process of scheduling his hours and was realizing
that he had promised to analyze more people than he could accommodate.[6]
For the American and Swiss patients he had set aside a total of 30 hours,
expecting that at least one would drop out by the time he resumed his work
in October. This, however, had not happened. Freud asked whether Kardiner would consider working with one of his trusted followers—Ferenczi,
Abraham, or Rank. Kardiner replied emphatically that he would not. Given
that no one wanted to drop out voluntarily, Freud said, he would have to
come to a decision in some other fashion. He himself did not mind taking
on extra patients, but his wife and daughter would not allow it. He told
Kardiner to come back the next day; there would be a meeting to which all
concerned analysands had been invited. Kardiner was very worried about
losing his chance of working with Freud. At three o'clock the next day,
Freud presented the anxious group with this solution:

> "Well, gentlemen, my daughter, my wife, and I have reached a con-
> clusion, which I hope will suit all of you. My daughter Anna made the
> best suggestion. Being something of a mathematician, she figured out
> that $6 \times 5 = 30$, and $5 \times 6 = 30$. So if each of you will sacrifice one hour
> per week, I can accommodate all of you." We all agreed, and that was
> the beginning of the five-hour week.[7]

Relieved that Anna's ingenious calculation assured everyone of a place, the Americans accepted the cut in hours gracefully—without failing to notice, however, that the English group (James and Alix Strachey, John Rickman) did not have to make such a sacrifice. Freud was an Anglophile and made no secret of it.

THE INITIAL PHASE

With the formal arrangements finally settled, Kardiner went to his first hour excited and without fear; he was confident that Freud would help him with the neurosis he had earned from his analysis with Frink. Paula, the maid, showed him to the waiting room, where he inspected books and various photographs. At the time of the appointment, Freud appeared at the door of the consulting room, shook his hand, and waved him to the couch saying, "You know what to do."[8] Kardiner began by giving Freud a detailed account of his family background and early childhood.

Kardiner grew up in an environment marked by extreme poverty and neglect. His father, a Russian Jew, had immigrated to the United States alone at the age of 28 when he was no longer able to make a living in his hometown. After trying his luck in different cities, peddling various goods, Isaac Kardiner eventually settled in Philadelphia, where his wife and five-year-old daughter joined him from Russia. Shortly thereafter, the family moved again, this time to New York City, where Abram was born. His memories of the first few years of his life were of hunger, cold, and deprivation. Not only were the physical conditions dismal, but the emotional atmosphere in the family was one of unhappiness and depression. Arguments between the parents were frequent, over sex as well as other matters, and often ended with Isaac beating his wife. As a young boy, Abram was terrified of his father and his violent outbursts.

From his mother, a depressed, hardworking, abused woman, young Abram felt distant. Mildred Kardiner was frequently sick and finally contracted tuberculosis from her long trips to pick up coal from various charities during the cold New York winters. She died in November 1894 when Abram was three years old. Her funeral accentuated the loneliness her son already felt, and each fall for many years following her death he became depressed. With his father at work and older sister in school, young Abram was left to his own devices for many hours each day. Half a year after Mildred's death, Isaac remarried. Abram liked his stepmother; although she had a temper and frequently criticized Isaac for his lowly economic and social position, she was able, nonetheless, to provide a sense of security and stability the family had never before felt. The young boy had her full attention—she was unable to have children herself and favored him over his sister. When Abram was between four and seven, his stepmother often took him to her bed, asking him to fondle and suck her breasts. He developed a passionate attachment to her, mingled, however, with fear and mistrust.

When Abram was three and a half, Isaac officially appointed him his mother's mourner. This required early morning trips to the synagogue each day to recite the *kaddish* prayer. Kardiner later thought that his father probably felt guilty for having treated his wife so badly and may even have felt responsible for her death. Abram was called upon to atone for his father's sins. Later, as an adult, he wondered whether the role of mourner had been thrust upon him too early in life, and he imagined that his later difficulty in identifying himself as a Jew had begun at this point.

Kardiner's early upbringing left him with little self-confidence and a sense of defeat. He told Freud that this attitude was partially due to an identification with his sister, an unhappy, meek girl who had been forced into the role of substitute mother. Like her, he did not do well in school and almost did not graduate from high school due to his difficulty with math. Freud commented in the first analytic hour that he thought Kardiner was identified with his natural mother. This remark surprised Kardiner, and he could not readily agree. Freud did not press the point, and Kardiner continued with his story.

Kardiner was finally able to overcome his inhibitions as far as his academic career was concerned. A driving force behind his ambition was his fear of becoming one of the social outcasts he saw in the streets; in achieving, however, he surpassed his sister and was consequently burdened with a great sense of guilt. Kardiner also spoke to Freud about some childhood phobias, one of which was a great fear of masks and wax figures, a reaction he had so far been unable to understand. His childhood terror of Indians, acquired from history books, and Italians, who lived in the same quarter as the Kardiners and did not like Jews, was more easily explained: It represented the sense of danger permeating the environment in which he grew up.

As noted, the arrival of the stepmother had a positive effect on the entire Kardiner family, including Isaac. She demanded obedience and submission from the children, qualities the young Abram had already identified as necessary for his survival. She also passed on to him a strict code of ethics:

> My stepmother was also my policeman, who reported to my father what my conduct had been. She would write on my forehead "good" or "bad" with her index finger, which made it visible for the whole world to see. . . . Many was the time I was threatened with abandon-

ment or being sent "over the water," meaning to the prisons on Randall's or Riker's Island. . . . Thus was obedience the guide to my early years. My submission was complete and absolute.[9]

Freud had listened to Kardiner's story without saying much. At the end of the session he asked:

"Did you prepare this hour?" I replied, "No! But why do you ask?" "Because it was a perfect presentation. I mean it was, as we say in German, *druckfertig* (ready to print). I will see you tomorrow." He shook my hand and I left, elated, feeling impressed with the idea, "I can really engage him." As I left, I could not wait for my next hour to begin.[10]

Kardiner continued giving his history in the subsequent hours. At the age of 20, having received a B.A. from the City College of New York, he enrolled in Cornell University Medical School, at his father's suggestion. He enjoyed his studies and did very well academically. Toward the end of his first year there, he fell in love with a librarian, K. They dated for several months until she told him, without warning, that she had accepted another man's proposal to marry. Kardiner was shocked and depressed; in fact, he was made suicidal by the unexpected news and dropped out of school.

Even though his relationship with the young woman had lasted only about a year and had been based more on fantasy than reality, Kardiner was not willing to give it up. He pursued K. persistently for a while, but she did not change her mind. The rejection devastated him, and he was unable to commit himself to any other woman for a long time. Years later, K. sent Kardiner a letter explaining that she could not feel anything for anyone and that her behavior toward him had therefore not been directed against him personally; it was not much of a consolation. In 1914, Kardiner, then 23, enrolled in a doctoral program in anthropology and philosophy at Columbia University, but after one year he decided to return to medicine. He graduated at the age of 26 with special honors and began an internship at Mount Sinai Hospital.

After Kardiner completed this account of his life, Freud, who had listened attentively and had not interrupted once, spoke:

"Your reaction to the breakup with K. was unfortunately, as they say, 'in the cards.' Her treatment of you was a repetition of your reaction to the death of your mother. It left you confirmed in your feeling of worthlessness, abandonment, and depression. However bad your reaction was, I can say to you—and let this be a guide to your future—You may be down, but you will never be out." I felt very much encouraged

by Freud's observation. I evidently had more strength than I gave
myself credit for. Freud gave me a much needed boost! [11]

After two years at Mount Sinai, Kardiner was not sure which
direction to pursue professionally. He was unable to find work as a
physician, and although he was interested in psychiatry, he found the idea
of working in state hospitals unappealing. One day he happened upon a
book that presented a theory of phobias and compulsions from a psychoanalytic point of view. The author was H. W. Frink, his former neurology
teacher in medical school. Kardiner decided to meet with Frink to find
out more about psychoanalysis; it seemed to him to be an intriguing and
novel approach to the treatment of mental conditions, one that could be
practiced privately. After talking to Frink, who encouraged him in the
pursuit of this new science, which he thought had a great future, Kardiner
decided to become an analyst.

Frink suggested that Kardiner first increase his general psychiatric
knowledge by working in a state hospital; in addition, he advised the
young doctor to undergo a didactic analysis with him. Kardiner followed
his advice. Thus, in his late 20s he began a residency at Manhattan State
Hospital and started seeing Frink three times a week in psychoanalysis.
At the time, Kardiner was enthusiastic but completely naive about
psychoanalytic theory and technique; he followed Frink's directions in
good faith. Before long, however, he was terrified, for one day, interpreting a slip of the tongue, Frink told him that he wanted his father to die
because he was jealous of his relationship with his stepmother.

Kardiner continued telling Freud about his analysis with Frink the
next day. He admitted that Frink's interpretation had devastated him and
that he wanted to terminate the treatment immediately. Nevertheless,
he stayed. During this time of psychological turmoil, Kardiner had a
dream that left him feeling depressed but whose meaning neither he nor
Frink could decipher. In the dream, Kardiner is in a basement that is
cluttered with old furniture; from a balcony three Italian men are urinating on him. The following day Kardiner had to attend a staff meeting in
which a black patient was discussed; the diagnosis was schizophrenia and
memory loss. Suddenly, Kardiner had the terrifying thought that he could
suffer the same fate. He excused himself from work and went to his room,
where he eventually fell asleep and had a second dream. In this one he is
having sex with his stepmother; at the point of penetration, it feels as
though he is tearing up something inside of her.

Freud asked for associations. The only thing that came to Kardiner's
mind was a story he remembered his father telling about Christ. In this
story, Jesus' claim to having supernatural powers is based on his ability to
fly. It is only a trick, however; his secret is a piece of holy scripture that

he has stolen and sewn under his skin. A high priest who knows Jesus to be a con man imitates the trick. He manages to fly even higher, and when he is above Jesus, he urinates on him. Jesus falls to the ground, his magical powers dispelled.

As for the Italians in the dream, Kardiner recalled, he used to fear them when young; they were reputed to be impulsive and violent. Freud suggested the following interpretation:

> "The cellar with the discarded furniture simply means a long time ago, when you were a little boy; things discarded are the past. The Italians were those you most feared. Three Italians equal one big Italian, your father. You felt small, humiliated, outdone by your father and belittled by him. What the amnestic Negro you saw in staff was, was a projection into the future of what you actually feared in the past. What you feared was therefore not what was going to happen but what actually had happened, and which you not only forgot, but feared to *recall*. And what you feared with Frink was that if he knew of your murderous intentions toward your father, he would withdraw his love and support, as you once feared your father would. And what you feared was the return of your sense of humiliation which devastated your childhood."[12]

The second dream, Freud continued, showed the degree of Kardiner's strength, persistence, and masculine prowess that helped him survive the great difficulties and dangers of his early years; he commented that Kardiner seemed to have "a lot of fight" in him.[13] Kardiner then spoke about the sexual aspect of his relationship with his stepmother, which he had justified to himself with the thought that she was not his real mother. This, Freud pointed out, was a very conscious manifestation of the Oedipus complex and related to his analysis with Frink.

> "The analysis itself merely opened up your old latent fears of abandonment and your inability to be assertive with your father. This was the conflict that was the issue in the Frink analysis; namely, how dared you to compete with the man whose favor and support you wanted, and who you were afraid would humiliate you if you disclosed your competitiveness with him—to displace him, especially with your stepmother."[14]

THE MIDDLE PHASE

Freud's interpretation of these two important dreams provided the outline for much of the material that was to be covered for the remainder of the analysis. He had already suggested (1) that Kardiner had created in his mind, with the help of internal censors, a positive image of his father that concealed some other, more disturbing, feelings, namely, his competition with him for his stepmother's love and attention, and (2) that Kardiner, knowing his father's potential for violence, must have felt that provoking his anger was a dangerous thing to do. Freud's reconstruction of his early emotional life, all within the first week of the treatment, left Kardiner in a state of shock. "He dismissed me with this. It was the end of the hour and I left in a very agitated and disturbed frame of mind. I was not prepared for anything like this. Having heard the interpretation of this enigmatic dream of the three urinating Italians, I was very bewildered by the proceedings."[15]

The night following this analytic hour, Kardiner dreamed of watch-ing several men dig a trench. Their activity disturbs him, and he begs them to stop, insisting that it will not be worth their while, that the only thing to be found there is an old rag—a prediction that, to his satisfaction, proves correct. In association to the dream, Kardiner remembered a Guy de Maupassant story in which a man picks up a piece of string without noticing a valuable necklace lying right next to it; when accused of the theft of the jewelry, he asserts his innocence, saying that he has only picked up a string. In a second dream that same night, Kardiner finds himself sleeping next to a very big cat that is lying still and indifferent. Freud thought the first dream confirmed that he had been on the right track with his interpretations the day before: "Well, apparently we hit something important here," he said. "In the first dream, you obviously don't want me to pursue your relationship with your father. You want the picture to remain as you retouched it, and so, in the dream, you tell me not to go digging up the past, I will not find anything important."[16]

Still not sure what Freud was getting at, Kardiner asked what could have motivated him to revise his father's image. Freud replied that in the first years of his life, until the arrival of his stepmother, he was terrified of his father, a feeling he wanted to forget. His solution was to suppress that memory and replace it with the picture of the man his father became later with the help of his second wife. Compliance and submissiveness, Freud continued, were his means of making sure that the early, angry father would continue to lie dormant. At the time of the analysis, Kardiner accepted Freud's interpretation. Later, however, he thought that Freud had missed the most important point:

> The man who had invented the concept of transference did not recognize it when it occurred here. He overlooked one thing. *Yes, I was afraid of my father in childhood, but the one whom I feared now was Freud himself.* He could make or break me, which my father no longer

could. By his statement, he pushed the entire reaction into the past, thereby making the analysis a historical reconstruction. . . . I was now afraid to have Freud discover my concealed aggression. I made a silent pact with Freud. "I will continue to be compliant provided that you will let me enjoy your protection." If he rejected me, I would lose my chance to enter this magical professional circle. This tacit acceptance on my part sealed off an important part of my character from scrutiny.[17]

Freud's interpretation had left the second dream unexplained. Kardiner could make nothing of it and asked Freud what he thought. The cat, Freud replied, was Kardiner's stepmother. Thinking about his relationship with his stepmother in more depth, Kardiner realized that he did not trust her entirely; he was not convinced that she would protect him, particularly from his angry father. In light of these associations, Freud's interpretation of the indifferent cat as his stepmother seemed to make sense. But Kardiner was uncomfortable with this implied criticism of the woman who had done so much for him, and he began to insist that he was also very grateful to her. His protest annoyed Freud, who told him that he was denying the way in which her behavior had been harmful.

> For the first time in the analysis, Freud raised his voice. "You are mistaken about your stepmother. While it is true that she gave you a structured environment, she also overstimulated you sexually and thereby augmented your guilt toward your father. You took refuge from this dilemma by fleeing into your unconscious homosexuality by way of identification with your natural mother. The basis for this was that you identified yourself with your helpless mother, for fear of identifying yourself with the enraged, aggressive father."[18]

Once again Kardiner was puzzled by Freud's words, this time with regard to his comment about homosexuality. He reasoned as follows: It was true that he had always envied women for seemingly having it so much easier than men, their responsibility in the family being restricted to domestic chores. Men, by contrast, were burdened with the difficult task of making a living—which, in the case of his father, looked like a frightening lot indeed. The fact that his father had managed, under the most adverse circumstances, to meet this challenge must have made him feel in early childhood extremely inadequate and weak by comparison. Thus, his envy of women was not so much a wish to be like them as it was a rejection of the male role. Moreover, against the argument of homosexuality it could be said that his identification with women had never affected his sexual desire for them. How was he to understand Freud's comment about unconscious homosexuality? Freud replied:

"By identifying himself with the mother, the child surrenders his identification with the father, thereby discontinuing his role as rival to the father. This guarantees him the continued protection of the father, thereby answering his dependency needs." "What can I do about this?" Freud's answer was, "Well, just as with the Oedipus complex, you come to terms with it. You reconcile yourself to it."[19]

In the night following this hour, Kardiner had a frightening dream about a mask. His associations brought back memories of his childhood phobia of masks and wax figures. When Freud asked what in particular it was about the mask in the dream that had scared him, Kardiner replied that it was its expressionlessness, its frozenness. He remembered other dreams in which he was looking into a mirror that did not reflect the changes of his facial expressions. "The first mask you saw was your dead mother's face," Freud said. Kardiner writes of his reaction to this interpretation: "Now, this idea sent shivers through me when I first thought about it, but the circumstantial evidence from this dream and the associations led to the striking possibility that I had discovered my mother dead, while I was alone with her in the house."[20] Upon his return to the United States Kardiner asked his sister what she remembered about the exact circumstances of their mother's death. Being a few years older, she was able to recall that, indeed, little Abram was alone with their mother at the time she died; when she came home from school she found her mother dead and her brother crying. Throughout his analysis Kardiner found Freud's intuition and his interpretations of dreams and associations brilliant to the point of being uncanny.

THE TERMINATION PHASE

For the ensuing months, the work of analyst and analysand remained focused on the interpretation of the Oedipus complex and unconscious homosexuality. In March, five months after the beginning of the analysis, Freud announced that it was time to begin preparation for their last appointment, which would be on April 1. Kardiner was shocked; he felt completely unprepared for such a sudden ending. At first he tried to change Freud's mind. With surprise he realized that they had agreed on the termination date initially. The memory of this was so completely erased from Kardiner's consciousness that it seemed as though he had never known about it. But there was another piece of distressing news. Not only did he find out that his analysis was coming to an end, but he now learned that Frink, from whom he expected help with his career back in New York, was returning to Freud for further treatment. Kardiner remarked that he found this unsettling. Freud reminded him of a statement he, Kardiner, had once made, namely, that psychoanalysis could not hurt anyone. Whenever Kardiner said something to this effect, Freud had been furious because it seemed to imply that psychoanalysis could not do much good, either. Freud now said, "Well, let me show you something."

> He took out two photographs. "One of these is Frink before analysis, and the other is after one year of analysis." I was shocked at what I saw. In the first photograph, he looked as I had known him. In the second, he was haggard, emaciated, and looked twenty years older. What neither Freud nor I knew at this time was that the drastic change in Frink was due not to the analysis but to other causes.[21]

At about the same time that Freud had reminded Kardiner of the upcoming termination, he asked him for "*ein bißchen Durcharbeitung*"—a little working through.[22] Kardiner was puzzled. He had no idea what he was expected to do and asked Freud to explain. But Freud's answer did not help much. "He said, 'Well, why don't you bring your childhood neurotic manifestations into your current life?' "

> I did not know at the time that this was the main job of analysis, but I did say to Freud, "I thought that was your job." However, at that time Freud didn't consider it to be so. He thought that once you had uncovered the Oedipus complex and understood your unconscious homosexuality, that once you knew the origins and the sources of all these reactions, something would happen that would enable you to translate these insights into your current life and thereby alter it. However, as for me, at the time his invitation . . . only left me bewildered. From this point on, the analysis drifted. In this period, I only remember having two dreams.[23]

The first dream was about a Russian winter landscape, which reminded Kardiner of the time following his mother's death when he had to wade through big mountains of snow on his daily visit to the synagogue, where he said prayers for her. Freud only remarked that the dream was depressive in nature and seemed related to his mother's death. The second dream was about the console of the organ at his former college, which he found facing one direction first, then another. In association to this dream Kardiner remembered a particular professor whose musical skills and recitals he had admired a great deal. Freud had no comment.

Against Kardiner's protestations the analysis ended, as planned, on April 1, 1922. Kardiner was not ready to leave, and Freud's insistence on keeping the termination date made him angry. In the last hour Freud signed a photograph upon request, but Kardiner was still disappointed.

We just chatted, I cannot remember about what, but when I was leaving, he said, "I wish you well and hope that someday you will have the good fortune to make a good marriage," and as a last word, "Someday you will be a wealthy man." I still do not know why he added that. I had been waiting for him to make some comment about the analysis, hoping, of course, that he would have glowing things to say, or that at the very least he would pull things together, sum it all up in some way. None of this happened.[24]

If Freud did not tell Kardiner himself what he thought of the analysis, he did mention to Frink in several letters that he was more than satisfied with the results. In fact, one letter read, "Kardiner's analysis is complete and perfect. He ought to have a great career."[25] Although flattered, Kardiner resented that Freud had not told him this personally.

Whatever the criticisms he had of Freud and whatever the anger left from the termination, Kardiner was, all told, more than happy with his analysis. He liked Freud a great deal; he found him friendly, humorous, direct, and personable. One time, when Kardiner observed aloud that he seemed depressed, Freud replied that he could not get over his daughter Sophie's death the previous year; he even invited Kardiner to visit his son-in-law and grandchildren in Hamburg on his way back to the United States. On another occasion, Freud asked Kardiner why he thought his daughter Anna could not find a husband; Kardiner answered that she probably could not find anyone capable of living up to the image of her father. At times, Freud liked to gossip about various members of the analytic circle, made jokes about psychoanalysis, or talked about his concern for the future. But Kardiner could not always be sure of Freud's mood.

He regarded it as his privilege to say to me one day, when I was discussing his theory of primal parricide [*Totem and Taboo*], "Oh, don't take that too seriously. That's something I dreamed up on a rainy Sunday afternoon." But then again, if you did not take it seriously, your head would come off. I didn't know which way it was. "Well," he would say, "this was just an idea"; but if you opposed him, you got into serious trouble.[26]

While Kardiner was in Vienna, a story circulated that illustrates the consequences a serious disagreement with Freud could have. It concerned a fellow American student, Clarence Oberndorf, who had brought a dream to his first appointment with Freud. In the dream Oberndorf is in a carriage pulled by two horses, one white and the other black. Knowing that Oberndorf had been raised by a black nanny, Freud interpreted the dream as an expression of so great an ambivalence about whether to choose a white or black woman that he would never marry.

This interpretation infuriated Oberndorf, and they haggled about this dream for months, until Freud got tired of it and discontinued the analysis. Freud was unequivocal in his condemnation of Oberndorf's character and of his ability, and later on he even refused to write a preface for a book he had written.[27]

Oberndorf never married.

Freud often spoke disparagingly about Adler and Stekel. Losing Freud's favor could be damaging to a psychoanalyst's career; after his aborted analysis with Freud, Oberndorf found himself excluded from a committee that was to reorganize the New York Psychoanalytic Society upon direct orders from Freud. On the other hand, when he liked someone, Freud could be lavish with praise. About Lou Andreas-Salomé he said, "There are some people who have an intrinsic superiority. They have an inborn nobility. She is just one of those people."[28]

Kardiner describes a directness and unpredictability about Freud that could be puzzling. Another American analysand of Freud's had begun an affair with a woman in Vienna while his wife was in New York. After the termination of his treatment, the wife came to Vienna unexpectedly to find out what her husband was up to. Suddenly the man became impotent. Panicked by this development, he made an appointment with Freud and told him what happened.

> He thought Freud would wring his hands and take him back into analysis. Instead, Freud did not utter a word during the entire interview, and when his hour was up, he rose, seized my friend's hand with the usual handshake, and said, "Und jetzt sehe ich dass Sie ein wirklich und [sic] anständiger Kerl sind" (Well, now I see that you are a really decent fellow!), and ushered him out.[29]

The entire group of Freud's American patients were so shocked and bewildered by this response that they called a meeting to figure out what Freud could possibly have meant.

Freud's analysands all knew each other. When comparing notes about their analytic sessions, it became apparent one day that Freud was behaving differently with Kardiner. This earned him an invitation to tea from the English patients.

> John Rickman said to me, "I understand Freud talks to you." I said, "Yes, he does, all the time." They [John Rickman and James Strachey] said, "Well, how do you do it?" I answered, "I don't exactly know. Maybe it's the hour of the day, maybe I keep him interested, maybe I keep hopping. I don't know, but he is quite garrulous. How is he with you?" They both said, "He never says a word." Rickman added, "I

suspect he sleeps. In fact, I know he does, because I know how to wake him. I just stop talking, and after a few moments of silence, Freud jumps in with a 'Yes, yes—go on, please.' One time I even said to him, 'What I said wasn't very important, Herr Professor, so you can go back to sleep.' "[30]

Rickman found his experience with Freud not very helpful. Kardiner wondered whether Freud's reticence with his British students might have been responsible for the tendency of analysts in the English school of psychoanalysis to speak very little during treatment sessions.

Kardiner thought his work with Freud inadequate from a training point of view but very helpful personally. As a result of the analysis, for instance, he felt less inhibited by his fears and conflicts—in particular, his conflict over being analyzed. Kardiner's criticisms of his analysis with Freud focused on the handling of the termination and the transference, Freud's insistence on the importance of unconscious homosexuality, and the lack of opportunity to work through conflicts in the analytic relationship. Kardiner once asked Freud how he regarded himself as an analyst. Freud replied, "I'm glad you ask, because, frankly, I have no great interest in therapeutic problems, I am much too impatient now." He continued:

> "I have several handicaps that disqualify me as a great analyst. One of them is that I am too much the father. Second, I am much too much occupied with theoretical problems all the time, so that whenever I get occasion, I am working on my own theoretical problems, rather than paying attention to the therapeutic problems. Third, I have no patience in keeping people for a long time. I tire of them, and I want to spread my influence."[31]

Kardiner disagreed. He thought Freud was a great analyst, brilliant and intuitive, with a special ability to stay close to the material at hand. Over 50 years later, Kardiner thought that the analysis had been one of the "peak experiences" of his life.[32]

Freud's Analysis of H.D.

Hilda Doolittle was born on September 10, 1886, in Bethlehem, Pennsylvania. She was the daughter of Charles Doolittle, a professor of mathematics and astronomy at Lehigh University, and his second wife, Helen (née Woole). The family moved to Philadelphia when Hilda was nine, and she was educated there at Friends Central School and later at Bryn Mawr College. H.D. left college during her second year owing to ill health and went to Europe in 1911, at the age of 25, ultimately making Switzerland her permanent home. Encouraged by Ezra Pound, her intimate friend and mentor, Doolittle became a leading figure in Imagist poetry, a movement that sought to free poetry from Victorian embellishment by conveying impressions directly through the precise and economical choice of words. She married another Imagist poet, Richard Aldington, in 1913.

In 1915, already emotionally estranged from her husband, H.D. met and developed an intellectual and romantic (although unconsummated) relationship with D. H. Lawrence. In 1918, at 32, H.D. entered a period of emotional crisis stemming from several critical life events: her brother was killed in the war; her marriage broke up; her father died; and she gave birth to her only child, Perdita (an earlier pregnancy had ended in abortion). Her great solace at this time, and for many years after, was a new, warm friendship with Winnifred Ellerman, whom H.D. called Bryher.

In 1925, Doolittle published *Collected Poems*, which established her reputation as a leading poet and was followed over a long career by numerous other creative works. She was the recipient of many awards and other honors, including the Award of Merit Medal for poetry from the American Academy of Arts and Letters, which was awarded shortly before her death. She died of a heart attack in 1961 at the age of 75 in Zurich, Switzerland.

Our presentation of her analysis is based on her book *Tribute to Freud* (1956) and on her correspondence with Bryher MacPherson. During H.D.'s stay in Vienna, she wrote almost daily letters to her friend, who was taking care of Perdita and the household in Switzerland. The correspondence is as yet unpublished and is quoted here in its original form (except for corrections of spelling and punctuation). When H.D. began her analysis with Freud, she was 46. Freud was 76.

Our account of H.D.'s analysis is much fuller than our account of Kardiner's. Indeed, she presents so much material and interpretation from the first week that it seems sufficient to fill an entire analysis. H.D.'s story has a dreamy fluidity that is apparently the authentic expression both of her particular sort of poetic gift and of a borderline personality relying upon dissociative splitting as a defense mechanism. What is interesting is how comfortable Freud seems in these waters, as though he is sailing along with his patient in a glass bottom boat, examining her descriptions of exotic fish and even contributing some of his own. Here again a stereotype of Freud is violated: Were his patients not all high-functioning hysterics and obsessives? Did he not insist that psychoanalysis is suitable only for the oedipally developed? With H.D., we see Freud learning more about the primacy of attachment to the mother in the girl's development and welcoming the new insight with scientific excitement. Clearly, he finds the maternal aspects of the transference at times unwelcome, yet he remains united with H.D. in a voyage of discovery. Despite many difficulties, analyst and analysand became, as H.D. told Bryher, "terribly en rapport and happy together."[1]

* * *

H.D. arrived in Vienna by train from Switzerland on February 28, 1933. She called the Freud residence immediately to find out the time for her appointment, but Freud was busy and later left a message saying that he expected to see her the following day, March 1, at five o'clock. H.D. had first contacted him in the winter of 1932 at the suggestion of Hanns Sachs, with whom she had had several analytic sessions.[2] Freud was agreeable to analyzing her but had postponed the starting date a number of times: At first he had no openings; then he, knowing her health was fragile, did not want her to travel in the dead of winter, especially when there was an epidemic of the flu in Vienna.

THE FIRST WEEK

On March 1, 1933, Hilda Doolittle made it to Freud's office and the family apartments at 19 Berggasse just in time for her appointment. She was nervous. She felt faint and cold and refused to give up her coat to the maid who was trying to make her feel comfortable. Freud suddenly appeared in the doorway of the waiting room and waved her into his office with the remark, "Enter, fair madam."[3] His kindly words did not alleviate her anxiety; she thought about leaving. She managed to focus her attention on Freud's art collection, which covered entire walls of the consulting room and adjacent study, and was further distracted by his dog, a chow who came to greet her. Still wrapped in her coat and avoiding the couch, H.D. began to talk. She spoke of her previous analytic experiences, in 1931 with Mary Chadwick in London for a total of 24 sessions, and in 1932 with Hanns Sachs in Berlin for several preliminary meetings; both of these had been unsatisfactory. Freud listened, then said he would prefer her to lie down. She wrote Bryher:

> He has a real fur rug, and I started to tell him how turtle [Sachs] had none, he seemed vaguely shocked, then remarked, "I see you are going to be very difficult. Now although it is against the rules, I will tell you something: YOU *WERE* DISAPPOINTED, AND YOU *ARE* DIS-APPOINTED IN ME." I then let out a howl, and screamed, "But do you not realize you are everything, you are priest, you are magician." He said, "No. It is you who are poet and magician."[4]

Freud pointed out that upon first entering the room she had preferred to look at the art objects rather than at him. But, protested H.D., she *had* made a connection with him; Yofi had welcomed her, and she took that to mean that Freud liked her, too. This reminded Freud of the saying "Love me, love my dog," which he, however, misquoted as "Like me and you like my dog." When H.D. corrected him, he apologized; it must be painful, he said, for someone, like herself, with a gift for language to listen to his bad English. But H.D. was still preoccupied with his observation that she had ignored him initially.

> [I told him] he was not a person, but a voice, and that in looking at antiquity I was looking at him. He said I had got to the same place as he, we met, he in the childhood of humanity—antiquity—I in my own childhood. . . . It was terrible. . . . He is not there at all, is simply a ghost and I simply shake all over and cry. He kept asking me if I wanted the lights changed. He sat, not at, but on the pillow and hammered with his fist to point his remarks and mine.[5]

H.D. began telling Freud about her background, and they discussed the war. At one point Freud observed that she was English from the United States and asked her what that made him. She felt compelled to reply that he was a Jew. Freud said, "[T]hat too was a religious bond, as Jew was the only member of antiquity that still lived in the world."[6] Toward the end of the hour, H.D. acknowledged, referring to the earlier part of their conversation, that perhaps she *was* disappointed to find that she was taller than he; her 5' 10" had always made her uncomfortable, and she did not want to be a grown-up in the analysis. Freud made her stand next to him to show her that even though she was taller, it was not by much. As she was leaving, Freud pointed out that she had left her bags on the couch. This slip, she thought triumphantly, proved that she was right after all: She was *not* disappointed, she wanted to come back.

H.D. had cried for much of this first meeting. She was terrified of Freud, who seemed like Oedipus Rex himself. She complained to Bryher that she had expected him to be quiet but here he had talked half the time, had not allowed her to fantasize and dream, had pounded on the couch with his fist. Freud's intense presence unsettled her. But the following day she discovered that he could be quite different. She was to say later that Freud had a hundred faces.[7]

The following day, March 2, Freud took H.D. to the adjacent room, his study, to show her some art pieces. He first picked up an ivory Vishnu from India, a figure that made H.D. uneasy by reminding her of the visions she had had many years before in Corfu. The visit to the sanctum, as she called it, impressed her deeply.

> This was not his favorite, this Oriental, passionate, yet cold abstraction. He had chosen something else. . . . "*This* is my favorite," he said. He held the object toward me. . . . It was a little bronze statue, helmeted, clothed to the foot in carved robe with the upper incised chiton or peplum. One hand was extended as if holding a staff or rod. "She is perfect," he said, "*only she has lost her spear.*" I did not say anything. He knew that I loved Greece. . . . I stood looking at Pallas Athené, she whose winged attribute was Niké, Victory, or she stood wingless, Niké A-pteros in the old days, in the little temple to your right as you climb the steps to the Propylaea on the Acropolis at Athens. He too had climbed those steps once, he had told me, for the briefest survey of the glory that was Greece.[8]

H.D. confessed that she had been overwhelmed the day before to find him surrounded by such a magnificent collection of classical art, art for which she had a passion, too. They engaged in an animated conversation about Greece, Egypt, and ancient myths. She told Freud about a dream in which a princess finds a baby in a basket. The dream inspired a discussion of the Moses saga, but Freud also interpreted its meaning in terms of her family history. It showed, Freud said, that she herself wanted to be Moses so as to be important and special to her mother, by whom she had felt rejected.

> He asked me again if I was Miriam or saw Miriam, and did I think the Princess was actually my mother? He said a dream sometimes showed a "corner," but I argued that this dream was a finality, an absolute, or a synthesis. Nor was I, as he had suggested in the first instance, the baby, the "founder of a new religion." Obviously it was he, who was that light out of Egypt. . . . But the Professor insisted I myself wanted to be Moses; not only did I want to be a boy but I wanted to be a hero.[9]

In this second hour H.D. mentioned her concern about the fact that she had not yet received the money for the analysis from Bryher.[10] Freud replied that this was not a problem since he did not accept advance payment; it was his custom to write up the bill at the end of each month.[11] After this appointment H.D. was happy, calmer; she felt right about being with Freud. There appeared to be a special connection between them based on their common interest in art and myths. It had already become obvious to her that being in analysis with Freud was regarded as a supreme privilege by the members of the intellectual community in Vienna; now, in addition, she seemed to be of special interest to Freud himself.

The ivory Vishnu Freud had shown H.D. reminded her of a fantasy or dream or real event—she did not know which it was—in which a very old man chooses her from among a group of children (she is the only girl) and allows her entrance into his garden. She may pick anything she wants from his garden. She selects what appears to be the only flower, a white Easter lily. She takes it to her mother, who plants it on the still-fresh grave of her grandfather. The old man then appears in a sleigh, and the two of them, covered by a fur rug, take a ride through the snow. When H.D. told Freud that she was not sure whether this story was based at all in reality or was entirely a product of her imagination, he replied that it did not matter because it showed how her mind worked. H.D. said that she had been very attached to her grandfather, who was a priest. Knowing that she had been born in Bethlehem, Pennsylvania, and had grown up in a house on Church street, Freud commented that the old man in the fantasy was clearly God. He had already said that he attributed great significance to her place of birth, in terms of the Christian myth, and now he asked her to say more about her religious background, which was Moravian.

H.D.'s description of a special candle ritual on Christmas, in which each person received a lit candle to carry home after the service, particularly interested Freud and inspired a lecture on the phallic significance of candles, as well as the comment that this early Moravian service captured the essence of true religion. H.D. was overwhelmed by his response. She wrote to Bryher:

> I was shattered and had some filthy dreams after all that exaltation, last night, but I look forward to today. It's all very uncanny, much more "magic" than I had anticipated, a collection of green and blue antique Greek and Crete-like glass jars in another case; there is so much I can't take it all in. He is like an old, old bird. He jerks out his arm, commandingly, like a terrific old hibou sacré. It scares me to death. . . . He keeps telling me to speak out what is on my mind, but I don't, just lie there and chirp to him (in my mind), "Little, old, old hibou. You are nothing but a little old, old owl."[12]

In terms of personality and interests, H.D. thought she most resembled her mother and maternal grandfather, both of whom were very creative and spiritual people. Her mother was from New England and was a lively, artistic woman who was in charge of a huge household. Her father, a withdrawn astronomy professor from Indiana, was engrossed much of the time in scientific research. One of his two sons from a previous marriage came to live with his second family, which included three more sons by his new wife and H.D., the third-born child and only daughter (two daughters had died in infancy). Knowing that her mother preferred an older brother and that she could never live up to her father's expectations of becoming a renowned scientist, H.D. felt like a failure as a girl and incompetent as a boy. After the hour on March 4 she found herself thinking that March 4 was her father's birthday, but then she suddenly realized that it was actually the date D. H. Lawrence had died. She did not mention Lawrence to Freud, even though he had reminded her of him immediately. She also thought of Freud as grandfather and called him Papalie in her mind.

In the next several hours H.D. told Freud in greater detail about the war period and the years following it. Two clusters of events had eventually combined to cause her breakdown, each one revolving around a pregnancy. The news of her first pregnancy arrived on the same day World War I was declared. She was 26 years old and had just gotten married. Although a baby had not been planned, she was looking forward to its arrival. When this pregnancy ended in a stillbirth—which she resentfully attributed to the shockingly abrupt announcement by her husband, Richard Aldington, of the news that the *Lusitania* had gone under with thousands of people aboard—she went into a deep depression.[13] The second pregnancy, in 1918 at age 30, resulted from a liaison with Cecil Gray, a man with whom she had become involved after finding out that her husband was having an affair. H.D. left both Gray and her husband and during her pregnancy fell ill with Spanish influenza, the cause of a dangerous epidemic responsible for many deaths. To her mind, it was nothing short of a miracle that both she and her daughter survived. Freud told H.D. that he remembered that season well, since his own daughter Sophie had died of the same disease. He then showed H.D. a locket, attached to his watch chain, in which he carried her picture.

While H.D. was surrounded by death and faced with the possibility that she and her child might die, she received news that her favorite brother had been killed in the war. A few months later her father died—from shock over the news, she felt. It was during this time that she met Bryher, an unhappy, wealthy woman eight years younger than herself. Bryher fell in love with her and promised to take her on trips to the Scilly Isles and Greece. In 1919, prior to her daughter's birth, H.D. also met Havelock Ellis, whom she admired greatly. Freud complimented her on her storytelling ability: "Ah, you tell this all so beautifully."[14]

Soon after H.D. gave birth to Perdita (at age 32), she went to the Scilly Isles with Bryher, but Ellis, who had lived and worked on his books in Cornwall for many years, was on her mind. This is when she had what Bryher later referred to as the "jellyfish" experience, a breakdown of ordinary consciousness into a kind of visionary state or trance that resulted, H.D. thought, from the traumas she had just experienced.[15] She felt as if she were under water, enclosed by a diving bell and a bell jar, one covering her from the top and one from the bottom; she could still see what was going on around her, but she felt somehow removed from that world. Bryher, whose presence H.D. believed helped inspire this fantasy, encouraged her to let it go on. H.D. was looking forward to telling Ellis about it, certain that he would be interested in the psychological aspects of her unusual state, but when she later showed him the notes describing what had happened, he seemed indifferent. Freud indicated that he understood the meaning of her experience and at the end of the hour asked her, with concern in his voice, whether she was feeling lonely.

Ellis had disappointed H.D., but she felt she could trust Freud. Telling him about the Scilly trip made her feel even more connected to him. She wrote Bryher toward the end of her first week in analysis:

> Have clicked like mad with papa, since embarking on the Scilly Isles and the Fish Notes. He looks a very wise old owl and shrugs with his left shoulder-wing and says, "Ach, later, I will explain all that—it is very simple." However, I must say he is an exquisite old fish-papa and

seems most excited over the life-in-myth that I seem to have had "pockets" of, what with Bethlehem, all the Greek cult and the fish experiences. He seems very interested in the Fido [Bryher] and its fido-mind.[16]

Freud told H.D. that he thought Bryher had intuitively understood what had happened in the Scillies. Bryher was quite present in the analysis—and not just as H.D.'s friend and benefactor. She established a correspondence with Freud and in the course of H.D.'s analysis sent him books, magazines, flowers, and donations for the psychoanalytic society. At one point H.D. showed him photographs of Bryher.

He looked at the pictures through a second pair of double lenses that he puts on, and said, "But surely I have seen that face? . . ." He turned to me and said, "But she is ONLY a boy." I think that rather wonderful; then he said, "But she looks like a northern explorer." So . . . there you are, all neat on the map. Is it not beautiful?[17]

Freud's comment about Bryher being "only a boy" gave rise to a dream in which H.D. was defending her little brother's adventuresomeness against their mother's criticisms.

H.D. was now very pleased about working with Freud. She found him wise, attentive, and sharp but also funny, informal, and obviously keen on gossip about Ellis. She felt they had much in common. In addition to their interest in art they both loved animals, and although dogs were not her favorites she was touched by Freud's obvious attachment to his chow, Yofi, who was present every hour and received much attention. From the beginning, H.D. was impressed with the unexpected turns her analysis would take; she never knew what was going to happen in the next hour. For instance, when she told Freud about the still-disturbing Scilly experience, he did not insist that she lie down. He surprised her in other ways—with comments, ideas, interpretations. One day he said that she had an interesting face but that he could not read it; this made her cry. Even though H.D. was now feeling safe, she began to realize that she was avoiding two topics: Lawrence and the atrocities that were being committed against Jews in Germany.

H.D. had a dream in which two women friends are arguing. One of them takes some boxes and jewel cases that belong to H.D. She defends her possessions passionately, as they have been given to her by her mother. The two women, H.D. realized when interpreting this dream, clearly were rivals for her mother's love. In further associations she recalled having felt betrayed by an uncle who had promised to show her a bear in the sky; there was no such creature there, only constellations of stars.

The Professor found me a thick rug now, for the couch. He always seems interested when I tell him of my animal findings and fairy-tale associations. At least, it was not my father who deceived me. The Professor said I had not made the conventional transference from mother to father, as is usual with a girl at adolescence. He said he thought my father was a cold man.[18]

This last comment made H.D. remember some nice things her father had done. But before long her thoughts once again returned to death and birth. It was in March, the same month she was now seeing Freud, that she learned of her father's death; it was also the month her mother died. On the other hand, March was the month in which both Lawrence and her daughter had been born. She kept thinking of Lawrence.

In another dream, first Ellis is the patient and H.D. the analyst, then vice versa; H.D. is concerned that Ellis will not be interested in psycho-analysis or understand her. In her associations H.D. remembered an accident her father had had when she was 10 years old, the cause of which remained a mystery. She had been extremely frightened, and she was worried that he might die. The memory of this incident was so traumatic that she repressed it for 35 years, until her analysis with Chadwick. Even now it scared her. And when she spoke of it to Freud, she carefully avoided elaborating the emotional terror related to it. In the following hour Freud told her that he could see "from signs" that she did not want to be analyzed.[19] She realized that he was right; she was afraid he would find out about her constant anticipation of disaster, presently in the form of the Nazis. Her thoughts, once again, returned to Lawrence. She was reminded of the man in Lawrence's last book who was buried alive. H.D. felt as though she were buried alive.

She dreamed about Lawrence looking the way he did in 1914, when they first met; he had reminded her of her father. In the dream he is surrounded by a group of children and a person who appears to be a secretary. The children stand around a piano, then change into ships. H.D. looks at one of Lawrence's books and is disappointed to realize that to her the psychology of his characters is not believable. Like Lawrence and her mother, H.D. had once considered becoming a teacher, but her free-association to the secretary in the dream brought up the memory that she had at one time worked in this capacity for her father. Her reaction in the dream to Lawrence's novel made her think of how envious she had always been of women who could unambiva-lently idealize men. She was certain Freud would not disappoint her but was constantly worried that death would end their relationship. She still could not talk about this fear. But Freud understood what was on her mind.

I did not know what enraged him suddenly. I veered round off the couch, my feet on the floor. I do not know exactly what I had said. . . . The Professor himself is uncanonical enough; he is beating with his hand, with his fist, on the head-piece of the old-fashioned horsehair sofa. . . . And even as I veered around, facing him, my mind was detached enough to wonder if this was some idea of *his* for speeding up the analytic content or redirecting the flow of associated images. The Professor said, "The trouble is—I am an old man—*you do not think it worth your while to love me*."[20]

H.D. was devastated. She answered that perhaps she was afraid. The fear of death was an important factor in all her relationships. Freud said later that the process of psychoanalysis itself was like death.

At this point only a little over a week had gone by in the analysis.

THE SECOND WEEK

H.D. wrote to Bryher of Freud's reaction when he noticed in one hour that she was checking her watch frequently:

Papa bit my tail almost off, O, so very, very delicately . . . He did not like me looking at my watch, but as his clock is in the corner at one's back, one has to. . . . One is not to see the time, one is not to look at ones watch. It meant all sorts of dire and diabolic things, on my part . . . that I was not really happy on his couch, that I really wanted him to die, that I really wanted to die myself, that I really did not believe the analysis would help me and so on. . . . my dear, I was a wreck. . . . Talk of the two-faced oracle of Delphi . . . Papa has a hundred.[21]

Freud then commented that any one explanation with a patient like her would not be sufficient, that there would always be multiple interpretations. H.D. left the office feeling sick.

About this time H.D. noted triumphantly that she had finally made the transference to Freud. To her disappointment, this had not happened with either Chadwick or Sachs. When she left a bottle of smelling salts on Freud's couch, he returned it to her the following day with the words, "This belongs to you—a little *green* bottle?"[22] She felt as though she had been caught. It is not clear what the forgotten smelling salts symbolized exactly nor how they elucidated the nature of the transference, but she and Freud now came to the following conclusion:

Chiron [Ellis], big and remote and dumb, is father-symbol and papa is sort of old Beaver. . . . Well, there is the language, of course, and his being small and delicate (woman) and having lots of friends and relatives (family, analysands) and so on. But papa was too sweet, when I told him of my constatation, he beat the pillow and said, "*But you are very clever.*" . . . He said he suspected it, then he said . . . "But—to be perfectly frank with YOU—I do not like it—I feel so very, very, very MASCULINE." He says he always feels hurt when his analysands have a maternal transference. I asked if it happened often, he said sadly, "O, very often."[23]

Freud and H.D.'s mother (referred to in the preceding passages as Beaver) were also connected in H.D.'s mind through their interest in art, but a dream about a cathedral, the analysis, and a united father and mother indicated to H.D. that the transference was not entirely maternal.

With the transference in better balance, H.D. could now finally talk about Lawrence. She had met him when she was 26 years old. It was the time of her first pregnancy and the outbreak of the war. Their relationship was intense and passionate but ultimately ended in anger. H.D. was fascinated by Lawrence's genius and intellectual power; he considered her a disciple. He loved and admired her for being gifted and cerebral but did not want her for a lover. They were like each other in many ways: Both were dreamers—perfectionistic, mystical, spiritual. Even though she worshipped him, in the end H.D. did not give herself up enough for Lawrence's taste. Her own strong personality stood in the way of total surrender. Lawrence ended up distrusting her, and after she left her husband to move to Cornwall in 1918, they did not meet again. Lawrence's reaction left H.D. feeling abandoned and betrayed; the disappointment stayed with her for a long time. Lawrence later denounced her completely, telling her in a letter that he hoped never to see her again.

In a dream about the smelling salts, H.D. throws salt on her typewriter. She interpreted that she was salting her "savorless writing with the salt of the earth, Sigmund Freud's last utterance."[24] Thinking about the books she had written, H.D. realized that she had never been entirely satisfied with her style, which seemed to her unemotional and cerebral. She recalled having read a statement by Freud that a woman could not be truly creative unless inspired by a man. H.D. had lost the supporters of her writing, Aldington and Lawrence. However, in Lawrence's last book, published after his death, she thought she recognized herself in the priestess Isis. It was a conciliatory gesture on his part, she thought. She had never talked about Lawrence to Chadwick, who, she felt, was unable to appreciate her creative mind. Sachs had suggested she continue her analytic work with a man, one superior to herself, perhaps even Freud? In a fantasy H.D. imagined herself a tiger.

This tiger may pounce out. Suppose it should attack the frail and delicate old Professor? Do I fear my own terrors of the present situation; the lurking "beast" may or might destroy him? I mention this tiger as a past nursery fantasy. Suppose it should actually materialize? The Professor says, "I have my protector." He indicates Yofi, the little lioness curled at his feet.[25]

H.D. dreamed about a mirror that in reality her mother had framed in velvet and painted with flowers. H.D. had very much admired it, as she had admired all of her mother's artistic creations. In the dream, Frances Gregg and Ezra Pound appear and both question H.D.'s enthusiasm about Freud. Freud comes through for her in this dream, saying that he could have helped Pound if he had known him. H.D.'s associations to the particulars of this dream made her wonder whether she disliked her books because they were too narcissistic. She wished she could have her mother's rich artistic ability. She recalled that she had met Frances Gregg when she, H.D., was in her early 20s, after she had dropped out of Bryn Mawr with failing grades and after separating from Pound; the women were in love and traveled to Europe together in 1911.

> When I told the Professor that I had been infatuated with Frances Josepha and might have been happy with her, he said, "No—biologically, no." For some reason, though I had been so happy with the Professor (Freud-Freude), my head hurt and I felt unnerved. Perhaps it was because at the end I tried to tell him of one special air-raid when the windows of our room in Mecklenburgh Square were shattered.[26]

Freud's interpretation of the dream was that H.D. was trying to avoid dealing with unpleasant memories and was leaving it up to psychoanalysis to resolve her conflicts.

H.D. returned to the memory of certain troubling experiences on her first trip to Greece, experiences she had never been able to fully explain. Most mysterious, perhaps, was what she referred to as the Van Eck episode.[27] Van Eck was a man she had met on the boat to Greece. There was flirtation between the two, a little romance. H.D. had been fascinated by this man: He was a worldly, educated, and witty individual among an otherwise dull group of fellow travelers. At one point, H.D. now told Freud, she went out on deck after a storm and found Van Eck there—or, at any rate, a man who looked like him. She could have sworn it was Van Eck, except that this man—to whom she referred as the Man on the boat—was taller and older and did not have Van Eck's visible facial scar. Freud expressed curiosity about how the story would proceed, but H.D. was still confused about the identity of the Man on the boat and unable to decide which part of her experience was real and which was not. The feeling of unreality quickly extended to other things: She now wondered whether the dolphins she thought she had seen when on deck with the mysterious man were real. Before long she began to question whether she herself was.

> I had read *The Centaur* a number of times, first in America. There was that same theme, that same absolute and exact minute when everything changed on a small passenger boat (as I remember) on the way to Greece. At an exact moment, the boat slipped into enchantment. So here, at an exact moment, by clock time, on an exact map, on the way to the Pillars of Hercules, on a boat that was bound for the port of Athens, there was a "crossing the line." I think in *The Centaur,* the narrator or hero knew the minute, the second that the line was crossed. I, the narrator of this story, did not know I had crossed the line.[28]

Even though Freud had said he was curious about the story, H.D. was frustrated and angry when he actually appeared more interested in Yofi, who was restless. She wondered whether he thought she was dramatizing the events. Freud asked if she had seen the man again after they parted in Athens. Yes, she answered, she had seen him twice—and he was not the Man on the boat.

In a recurrent dream, H.D. finds herself moved out of her hotel room by an angry landlady who tells her there is no space for her. With some difficulty she transfers her belongings to a hotel on the other side of the river, where her mother and Bryher are staying. Her mother says that she is only safe on this side. The dream had a nightmarish quality for H.D. and stirred up memories of a trip to Florence with her parents in 1912 as well as another visit there in 1919 during her second pregnancy. The dream also made her think of death: her mother's death and the influenza she had contracted when expecting her baby. Her own life and that of her child were in danger; at the time people were dying of it in the nursing home where she was staying. In fact, she recalled, when Bryher came to visit, the landlady asked her who was going to pay for the funeral in case H.D. died. She told Freud about it the next day, but he was still preoccupied with the Van Eck story.

> He asked first of Van Eck—was it an Austrian name? He said, "I have an idea." He rushed off and brought back a leather case and showed me the name, stamped inside the folder. It was *Vaneck.* He was interested to hear that Mr. Van Eck was the adopted son of the Victorian painter. He asked of the nationality.[29]

H.D. told Freud that it was difficult to recreate what had happened with Van Eck because in a way it had been just an ordinary romance. Freud asked how she understood the dream. In light of the memories it had brought up, she thought it might be about her fear of being moved when pregnant or her fear of dying. She recalled other times during the war when she had to move so as to be close to her husband, including one time in particular when she got lost at night. A stranger had offered her his room. Freud said that he knew who the bad landlady was—himself. H.D. objected to this interpretation, recalling that she had been angry at Chadwick, who thought she liked to talk too much. But Freud pointed out that Chadwick was only a "forerunner" of himself. Again H.D. protested, saying that there was no comparison between the two of them.[30] Freud asked for more history associated with the fear of being moved out. In response, H.D. recalled a trip with her parents during which she actually found her things transferred without warning to another room. Even now, H.D. acknowledged, every time she went back to her hotel she half expected to find that she was being moved out. The only other anecdote she could provide was being sent out of the room when she was naughty.

THE THIRD WEEK

Little more than two weeks had gone by in the analysis. During this time H.D. had been keeping a notebook in which she recorded her thoughts, memories, and associations. Freud told her, and repeated this several times in the following weeks, that he did not want her to prepare in any way, that he wanted their work to be spontaneous. H.D. also wrote almost daily letters to Bryher, many of which contain detailed descriptions of her relationship with Freud. Freud discouraged this also. Telling herself that the notes were not in preparation for her hours, H.D. kept up her journal for a while. After the second week she was, however, less revealing in her letters to Bryher, limiting her accounts of the analysis to the more mundane aspects. Freud was not against her reading psychoanalytic literature. In fact, he invited her to borrow any books she wanted from the library in his waiting room.

It was the middle of March now. Bryher and Perdita were getting ready for a visit to Vienna. H.D. was looking forward to seeing them both, but asked Bryher to wait so that the transference could really take hold. "I think I was right about this business getting Freud ALONE and STRAIGHT," she wrote, "as you see I made this peculiar, unexpected dip or drop into earliest layers, with mother-transference, which Freud says is most important."[31] From the beginning Freud had emphasized the importance of the conflict in her relationship with her mother and therefore the maternal transference, even though H.D. herself seemed to associate him more with her father, grandfather, and Lawrence. Freud told her that she had come to Vienna to find her mother (who had spent her honeymoon in Vienna) and pointed out the connection between her passion for Greece (*Hellas*) and her mother, whose name was Helen. In fact, he made her relationship to her mother the focal point of the analysis.

H.D. now continued with her story, starting at the point where she and Van Eck parted ways in Athens. Ellis, who had been with them on the boat, returned to London after a while, and H.D. went with Bryher to Corfu. Here she saw a series of pictures projected on a wall of a hotel room, pictures she believed to be important visions, a psychic phenomenon. Freud was very interested in these pictures and commented that her problem was "more subtle, more intricate than he had at first imagined."[32] He repeated that she should not prepare for her treatment hours. H.D. said she did not—and continued writing her notes. What had happened on Corfu was perhaps the most troubling of all the mysterious events from that time period. With Freud's help, she thought, she would finally be able to translate the puzzling symbols into personal meaning. Already, with his assistance, she had solved the mystery of the "jellyfish experience" on the Scillies: She told Freud it must have been some kind of prenatal fantasy. Freud replied, "Yes, obviously; you have found the answer, good—good."[33]

H.D.'s usual appointment with Freud was at five o'clock, her favorite time of day because of the pleasant memories it evoked of the British tea ritual. When Freud announced now, three weeks into the analysis, that he possibly needed to change the time of her session because a well-known patient of his, Mrs. Burlingham, was planning something for her, H.D. was shocked. She did not like being surprised in this fashion and worried that the change was going to be permanent. It did not help that "the Burlingham" had something to do with it; H.D. envied her closeness to Freud. At that point, however, nothing actually came of this proposal to change her treatment hours. But when the same woman a little later asked her directly whether she would exchange her Friday appointment time on a regular basis, H.D. agreed to it. On one other occasion Freud conveyed the request for a schedule change from another patient, J. J. van der Leeuw, a man from South Africa, whom H.D. sometimes encountered on the steps to Freud's house. Freud introduced the two analysands in the garden of his summer residence and let them arrange the matter between themselves.

When H.D. began to discuss seriously the "Writing on the Wall," as she liked to call the pictures in Corfu, Freud asked her a number of detailed and specific questions. He wanted to know their size, at what time she saw them, what kind of light there was in the room, and whether there were shadows. They were most certainly not just shadows, H.D. replied; in fact, the first figures or shapes looked as though they were drawn on shadow with light. The first image looked like a soldier; then there was a goblet or chalice, then a tripod. H.D., baffled by this sight, told Bryher what she was seeing. With Bryher's encouragement she let the vision continue. At the base of the tripod she saw a number of very small, black people, outlined in shadow. Whereas the first pictures had appeared complete, the following images were drawn right before her eyes as if by an invisible hand. A series of lines formed into a ladder. There was one last figure: Niké, the goddess of victory, was moving up from the last step of the ladder as if toward the wall. A number of broken curves, forming half-Ss, looked like question marks. Niké moved through a group of tent-like structures. H.D. believed later that these images were an oracle-like vision of the coming war.

> I thought, "Niké, Victory," and even as I thought it, it seemed to me that this victory was not now, it was another Victory; in which case there would be another war. When that war had completed itself, rung by rung or year by year, I, personally (I felt), would be free, I myself would go on in another, a winged dimension. . . . The picture now seemed to be something to do with another war, but even at that there would be Victory. Niké, Victory seemed to be the clue, seemed to be my own especial sign or part of my hieroglyph.[34]

To demonstrate what the last figure had looked like, H.D. took Freud to his study and showed him the painting of Niké on one of the Greek vases. Freud asked whether the experience had frightened her. No, she replied, but she was worried that Bryher might be afraid for her. Of all the stories H.D. had told him, Freud said, he found this one to be the most compelling and possibly dangerous. He added that he would not stop being fascinated with the human mind if he lived another 50 years.

When H.D. arrived for her next hour, Freud said that her Corfu experience had made him "think very hard."[35] She talked about some statues in a house in Cornwall that Lawrence had mentioned to her; asked what they were, she recalled an Osiris, Iris, and a mummy-owl. Freud invited her to his study, an excursion H.D. loved. She wrote to Bryher:

> He took me into the inner sanctum . . . to show me some more of the Egyptian images. I should think he had some hundreds, rows and rows AND rows. We had about half the hour sitting and talking over the Egyptian, I suppose this is part of the "treatment," anyhow, it is most thrilling and unexpected and links the whole thing up with Egypt, Crete, Greece.[36]

H.D. remembered an occasion when she had acted out what she referred to as "Indian dance-pictures" to cheer up Bryher, who was in a somber mood. In her opinion this was "some form of possession,"[37] but Freud disagreed.

> The Professor said, "It was a poem-series; the acting was drama, half-motivated by desire to comfort Bryher and neither 'delirium' nor 'magic' " . . . The Professor repeated, "You see, after all, you are a poet." He dismissed my suggestion of some connection with the old mysteries, magic or second-sight. But he came back to the Writing on the Wall. The drama, as he called it, he said held no secret from him; but the projected pictures, seen in daylight, puzzled him. . . . He said this was possibly a "symptom of importance."[38]

Freud allowed H.D. her preoccupation with magical and spiritual matters and her preference for interpreting her own experiences from that point of view, but he invariably showed her the connection between these supposed supernatural events and ordinary family conflicts. He reminded her again not to take notes of matters related to her psychoanalysis.

Through the American and English newspapers, H.D. was following the worrisome political situation. She still could not talk about it to Freud and failed to mention it as one of her associations to the following dream: The entrance to her house is barred by a man and a boy who seem threatening. Terrified, she calls out for her mother. Looking up to her flat, she sees her mother standing in the window with a lit candle in her hand. Her fear is gone.

H.D. told Freud of her disappointment on a recent trip when she could not land on Crete due to the weather conditions. Freud, too, loved Crete. "The Professor," she wrote Bryher, "said that we two met in our love of antiquity. He said his little statues and images helped stabilize the evanescent idea, or keep it from escaping altogether."[39]

While discussing the art of Crete, H.D. found out that Freud did not have a particular statue of a snake-goddess. When she offered to get one for him, Freud doubted that she would be able to. In a letter to Bryher, H.D. half jokingly comments that finding such a statue is now going to be her new goal in life. She was very enthusiastic in her description to Bryher about how well things were going: "We are terribly en rapport and happy together."[40]

THE END OF THE FIRST MONTH

Freud continued interpreting the material from H.D.'s treatment sessions, including her relationship with Bryher, in light of a mother fixation. He told her that both boys' and girls' initial attachment is to the mother but that in normal development girls transfer their affection to the father; this was, he said, a piece of psychoanalytic theory that had only recently been understood.[41] It was Freud's impression that H.D. had not achieved this last developmental stage, in part perhaps because her father had been somewhat cold. She wrote in her journal:

> The Professor said he thought my dance-dramas at Corfu were really a sort of display or entertainment for my *mother*. Did your mother sing to you? I said she had a resonant beautiful voice but that she had some sort of block or repression about singing. Our grandmother loved me to sing to her. . . . My older brother and I sang little nursery songs to our mother's accompaniment. The Professor said this held together. "It will simplify out, even more." I told him again that my mother died in spring, at this very time, and again I remember that Lawrence died too, in March.[42]

It was reassuring to H.D. that the discovery of this kind of fixation, as Freud told her, had only recently been made. It meant that it would not have helped her to be analyzed much sooner, as she sometimes wished. Freud said that she had become fixated at the earliest preoedipal stage; that her interest in the sea, islands, and Greece was symbolic of a "back to the womb" phenomenon; and that the Corfu pictures were the desire for reunion with her mother. H.D. agreed. She had always felt something was missing when Chadwick had spoken of her strong attachment to her father:

> Even Turtle [Sachs] said I was deeply attached to my father which I suppose I was and am, but I always felt there was a catch. . . . My triangle is mother-brother-self. That is, early phallic-mother, baby brother or smaller brother and self. I have worked in and around that, I have HAD the baby with my mother and been the phallic-baby, hence Moses in the bull-rushes, I have HAD the baby with the brother, hence Aldington/Cecil Grey, Kenneth, etc. I have HAD the "illumination" or the back to the womb WITH the brother, hence you and me in Corfu (island = mother), with Rodeck as a phallic-mother.[43]

Freud showed H.D. a letter he had received from Bryher and mentioned that she had also sent a donation to the psychoanalytic society of which he was very appreciative. They spent half the hour talking about Bryher and the increasingly difficult political situation. Although Freud had previously not shown his concern about it, he acknowledged that it worried him. If H.D. had not wanted to discuss this topic before because it was too upsetting, she now found it a waste of time to talk about outside matters. She had had a familiar nightmare the night before: In the dream she is traveling on a train with her daughter and a friend. An official in uniform searches her bags and finds several bottles of alcohol. He tells her and her companions to follow him. They seem lost on their way down some stairs. There is danger.

Freud asked for her associations, but the only thing that came to mind was a fear of being caught. Perhaps she was feeling guilty about something, Freud suggested. H.D. then realized that she had many memories related to trains. She described a trip from England to France, which stood out because she felt so relieved to have escaped. Freud complimented her again on her ability to tell stories.

> The Professor said, "You tell it all so beautifully." Before I leave, I fold the silver-grey rug. I have been caterpillar, worm, snug in the chrysalis. The Professor touches the little bell to warn the maid that this last analysand is about to leave. His elbow concludes its bird-wing dismissing gesture. The Professor says, "We have gone into deep matters."[44]

H.D. gave Freud some books Bryher had sent, which included one on chows. He showed the picture to Yofi, who at one point during the analytic hour, when Freud coughed, got up to lick his hands for a full five minutes. Freud apologized, then went on to press H.D. about her relationship with Ezra Pound, whose name had come up in the context of a dream. H.D. had been briefly engaged to Pound in her first year of college; he had broken it off in pursuit of another relationship. But he continued to support her creative endeavors and helped her get established in the London poetry circle. H.D. thought Freud was rather distant in this hour, very much in contrast to the previous one. In fact, she felt criticized after telling him how flattered she had felt two years before by the courtship of a man much younger than herself; Freud's response—"Was that *only* two years ago?"—sounded to her as though he thought at 46 she was too old for this kind of thing.[45] He also expressed surprise that she was 19 at the time of her first serious love relationship, the affair with Pound: "As late as nineteen?"[46]

With some reluctance, H.D. returned to the Van Eck story. After her arrival back in England from Greece, she had received a note from him with the request to forward an enclosed letter to his cousin. In H.D.'s mind, the question of whether this man was real or not was still not settled, and when the cousin, to whom she had sent the letter along with some of her poetry, did not answer, she finally decided that Van Eck was just a product of her imagination. However, several years later, she told Freud, she met the sister of this cousin, who confirmed his existence. It occurred to her to look Van Eck up in the London telephone directory. When she called the number listed there, someone asked whether she wanted to talk to Mr. or Mrs. Van Eck. She was shocked: The possibility that he might be married had never occurred to her. Bryher suggested that the thought was so disturbing because it reminded her of feeling betrayed by her husband. But H.D. still could not get Van Eck out of her mind. She found another phone number listed under his name and this time spoke to a man called Van Eck. Since he came to see her, she concluded that her fellow passenger on the boat to Greece must have been Van Eck, even though she was not sure she would ever have recognized him. With Freud's help, H.D. realized that there was a connection between Van Eck and her mother's brother, a talented young musician. There was one final chapter in the Van Eck saga. Some 10 years after the reunion in London, H.D. received the news that he was going to be ordained as a priest. Freud told her his thoughts on this:

> [T]hese details only confirmed him in his first impression, or opinion, that the Van Eck episode or fixation was to be referred back to my mother. The maternal uncle, church, art. The Professor asked me if I had ever wanted to go on stage. He said he felt I narrated these incidents so dramatically, as if I had "acted them out" or "prepared" before coming to him. I told the Professor how I loved "dressing up." . . . The Professor said he felt some sort of "resistance."[47]

Once again, Freud asked her whether she was preparing for her sessions. He repeated that she should discontinue her notes because the work needed to be spontaneous. It was not until then, a month into the analysis, that she finally followed his advice and stopped her daily journal entries. In her hours she continued talking about Crete, Freud's favorite Greek island; she even gave him some books on the subject. But Freud was now getting stricter about limiting their conversations to topics related to her analysis. H.D. surmised that he was trying not only to keep her on track but to curb his own desire to talk. She complained to Bryher, "Now he is scolding me for not being eager enough to do analysis and that I begin later and always end before time, and it is an 'indication' of resistance, so I have to go careful with 'dirt' outside legal matters of ps.a."[48]

Not only did Freud want H.D. to focus more on her own person, but he also thought she had spent enough time on the subject of the war years. She wrote in the same letter:

> I get a worse trauma about R.A. [Aldington], you must help me with it, as papa says now I have gone over all the historical war and post-war matter and he wants me to stick back in the child-period of pure mother fixation. He more or less gave me his blessing and forgiveness and dispensation for all past "sins," said it was not really necessary to dwell on all that, only as an indication of guilt toward mother, that

otherwise there was nothing "wrong," or words to that effect. The result was that I came home with a ghastly cramp and could hardly eat. I slept in the afternoon . . . I suppose it's getting back to the nursery.[49]

H.D. seemed to believe that her problems had to do with the fantasy of having a "magic phallus."[50]

Freud and H.D. left the Greek trip behind for the time being and talked about her acting. Freud told her he thought her mostly repressed desire to be an actress was the key in understanding her trouble with writing. Even though she found Freud's observation depressing, she had to agree.

H.D. was content with the progress she was making in the analysis, but she was beginning to feel quite homesick. At this time Bryher suggested that she might consider working with Freud for another three months at a later date, perhaps in the fall. H.D.'s response to this offer was mixed; she was happy with the analysis but found it difficult as well. Moreover, she already felt indebted to Bryher for financing the current period. In a passing comment she mentioned that she and Freud were now talking about sexual matters.

THE SECOND MONTH

On March 30, 1933, Bryher came to visit; Perdita and another friend followed a little later. It is difficult to tell what happened in the analysis during the first two weeks of April, since H.D. had discontinued her notes and the correspondence was interrupted for several weeks. Also, her letters to Bryher were now less revealing about the content of her sessions with Freud. When H.D. was alone again in Vienna, she wrote to Bryher, "I think now, I have had time to think, that papa smelt with the whisker that you and I had been chewing things too much. . . . I will write everyday details and so on. I do hope papa isn't going to bully me now."[51] Freud, incidentally, visited with both Bryher and Perdita during their stay.

Toward the end of April, H.D. made some comments about another writer and then described how Pound had helped her with the publication of her first poems. Freud said he was surprised that it had taken her almost a month and a half to make more than superficial comments about her writing. He attributed this to her modesty, but H.D. told him there was more to it. In the meantime, she was feeling much calmer. Freud shared this impression and pointed out that her dreams were unusually clear and showed "a state of harmony and inner satisfaction that is very significant."[52] He told her that she had a "rare type of mind he seldom meets with, in which thought crystallizes out in dream in a very special way."[53] The compliment scared her.

While things unconscious were calming down, the environment was getting more restless. Freud's 77th birthday was coming up on May 6, and so was the move of the entire Freud household to their summer residence just outside of Vienna. Since Grinzing was easily accessible by tram, the move did not affect the continuation of H.D.'s analytic hours. But the change frightened H.D. nonetheless. "Am much upset," she wrote her friend, "in the unconscious over the move of papa, contemplated in a week, to the 'country.' . . . It's very upsetting, but as last night I almost died, and yesterday told him I would rather go to London or Athens than to the 'country,' I have come to the conclusion that it is some dire birth phobia."[54]

In a dream H.D. had at this time Freud gives her a paper bag of sweets that she takes to a child whose name is Saint Margaret. Her associations revealed her jealousy of Mrs. Burlingham and the symbolic meaning of the paper bag as a uterus. H.D. concluded that the dream was a fantasy or a fear of becoming pregnant by Freud.

Indeed, there was a pregnancy in the Freud house. H.D. had found out in the middle of March that Yofi was pregnant. The very day after the aforementioned dream, H.D. wrote Bryher that she was afraid Freud might offer them one of the puppies, for he had asked her whether they had a garden in Switzerland, how many dogs were there, and so forth. After her next appointment she told Bryher:

> The worst has happened. . . . Papa has offered us one of Yofi's pups. What will we do about it? . . . [H]e wants the pup to have a garden and so on. He says, "We of our circle, have decided that it would be best to offer one of the puppies to Perdita." Now I do not think that "our circle" has anything to do with it, and I do think we better keep the puppy in our own hands . . . this will be a delicate little creature, very esoteric, and more our cup of tea. But, but, but . . . I do not want the responsibility so said *if* the puppy were strong enough to make the trip! Yes. He said at once that the puppy would be by the time I went and so on, and I am to have a special seance with the old dame on that farm. . . . It's just too Gawd-awful. . . . Fido, why have you gone and got me in this awful mess? I feel pregnant. . . . Please write, *don't* wire Freud "yes" as I am not sure it would be feasible. . . . O, please, I feel so very about-to-deliver.[55]

The next night H.D. had dreams about the puppy, dreams in which it was associated with death and impregnation. The question as to what to do about the puppy preoccupied her for a long time. She was flattered by Freud's offer but not sure she really wanted a dog. The thought that Freud might find out about her mixed feelings made her anxious, and she managed to avoid giving a definite answer until the matter finally settled itself. In the meantime, she continued to feel pregnant. Freud asked her for names of goddesses for the new dog.

THE THIRD MONTH

It was now the end of April. H.D. was homesick, and the possibility of extending her stay past June seemed unbearable. At the outset Freud had offered her a little over three months for the treatment; now he thought *she* had imposed this limit. When she reminded him that this was not the case, he let her know that she could stay on. She was again flattered; Freud must like me, she thought. But now that he and Bryher both were allowing for more time, H.D. was not sure she really wanted it; she felt "sick of psychoanalysis . . . battered . . . and sick for you all."[56] She considered Freud's upcoming birthday and the move to Grinzing a turning point, after which she would get ready to go home. A long and important dream described below indicated the beginning of a new phase; "the back of the analysis" was broken.[57] Nevertheless, H.D. remained unsure about whether to continue, telling Freud one day that she would stay as long as he would keep her.[58] Her concern about Freud's birthday and the question of what to give him were put to rest when he made it clear that he could not accept a present while the analysis was going on. Her stomach cramps, which she related to the pregnancy fantasy, continued. It was understood now that she was going to take one of the puppies.

The aforementioned dream, Freud thought, was related to her desire to end the analysis. The dream had a preface: H.D. is on a boat during a storm and tries unsuccessfully to play piano on deck. Bryher and Perdita are there. Another, smaller, boat with a number of women on it topples over. Freud's interpretation of this part of the dream was that it contained elements of both birth and death; perhaps the fear of death in birth. Freud had told H.D. before that thoughts of death could be expected to preoccupy her because of his age and because of the fact that both her father and brother died while she was pregnant with Perdita.

The dream continues with Bryher telling H.D. that she will take H.D. to meet a young, exiled prince who lives in a dark, empty place. The two women are now walking down a country lane; there are trees and a river. Bryher is dressed stylishly (unusual for her) in green and is outfitted with gigantic, precious pearl earrings, which then turn into less demonstrative moonstones. She tells H.D. she is wearing the earrings because a man by the name of Marcel likes them. They are now standing near a river, but the prince is not there. Bryher tells her that he did not want to be an exiled prince any longer and that he is now working on a farm or estate. In the darkness the river throws long shadows out of which emerge a herd of bulls and, with them, the prince. The bulls are quite unlike their real-life equivalents; they are small and friendly. Bryher introduces H.D. to the prince, and all three enter a house, where they sit together with an artist couple. Then H.D. finds herself in another room; someone is sleeping on a bed. She looks at herself in a mirror and notices that she is naked: "As I look at myself I am surprised to see that my front is like my back, only that it is smaller, the mons-Venus, a tiny replica of the buttocks, I am entirely smooth, like a child."[59] She likes the idea of being a virgin with two backs and thinks the mirror must be magic. However, not wanting to wake the sleeping person, she leaves and finds herself in another room, again fully dressed. This room looks Victorian and is cluttered with many small items, which make her wonder whether there will be a church sale. There are two Siamese cats and H.D. is worried that Bryher might get her one of them; she remembers two kittens once tearing up her house. She moves on to another scene. She sees railroad tracks going through a tunnel. The leader of a group of workmen tells her that she has to get on a train in order to pass through the tunnel. He helps her board it but seems discontent with the tip she gives him. She then gives money to the train guard but worries about whether he will think it is a tip or payment for the ticket. After getting off the train she finds her daughter, two years old, in the care of her mother and aunt. The child is dressed in white, the two women in black. It seems that she fights with the women, who seem to disapprove of her, over her daughter. She leaves the house. She gets on another train, but this time the guard is friendly. He offers her a paper, and she wonders whether it will be a "left" or "right" paper. To her satisfaction it is "white," meaning "right." She finally arrives in Vienna, her destination. Bryher is there and asks Freud whether he will eat with them in a fancy restaurant on his birthday; to H.D.'s surprise he and his wife, who will wear a new hat, will come. H.D. is now worried about how to carry on a conversation with Freud's wife in German.

H.D. and Freud worked on the interpretation of this dream for many days. There was no doubt about its significance in either's mind. A dream of the subsequent night, about a brown beetle, provided the clue to the interpretation. H.D. had been reading about astrology and in that context understood the beetle to represent her father.

> The clue is the fear and dread of Scorpio, my father, a cold, distant, upright, devoted father and husband for whose profession I had only terror, a blind fear of space and distances of the planets and fixed stars. . . . Scorpio grew wings in my dream. I ran forward across the floor to

open a door so that this deadly insect might run out. But as I open the door, he . . . flies into the branches of a small tree. . . . We have not interpreted this finally, but it is obvious that the fear is removed, the mystery, the glamour remains and is now recognizable in my reading and romantic interpretation of star-values which my father measured with cruel and exquisite accuracy, with a cold hermit logic and detachment.[60]

Freud told her he thought the bulls represented the "fat" years, the river perhaps the Nile. He himself, the prince, appeared as Joseph, the dream interpreter for the King of Egypt. Freud was pleased with this image in particular but liked the dream as a whole, telling her, "I keep on seeing more and more beauty in it."[61] When H.D. told him that the bulls were sacrificial white bulls, Freud quoted from Heine, "The oxen tremble," meaning a great discovery had been made. H.D. thought the river might be the Milky Way and that the bulls were also "mother-bulls." However, the most important part, both she and Freud agreed, was that the bulls/cows stood for her wish to get pregnant by Freud, who is fa-ther/mother. She associated the man to whom she gave a small tip with her first husband; the man who led her through the tunnel to a new life with Cecil Gray, the father of her daughter; and the man to whom she gave no money (i.e., did not have sex with) with Van Eck. H.D. under-stood Bryher in the fancy green outfit and pearls to stand for the woman, or moon, whereas Freud, the prince, was the sun.

> Maybe father and mother, but the father and mother each take attributes of the other, it is the mother-bull and the father-cow, all this too, works out with Egyptian symbolism. The trio is you, Freud, me (and a child). I gave tired and dreary feelings, all pregnancy, I now imagine. . . . Apparently, too, the little-dog represents a child, though he did most carefully present it to Perdita, I took it to be "ours," yours and mine. But this about the dog, oddly, came after the dream, about the second day of it, so fortunately I had the dream first.[62]

Bryher kept sending things for Freud: a book with Chinese names for the new puppies, a box of narcissus flowers. Freud liked the narcissus a great deal but told H.D. that his favorite was the gardenia.

> "This is almost my favorite scent, almost, if not quite, my favorite flower. It is the poet-narcissus." He went on to sobbing over the box, just such had grown all around their little house at Aus-see (?) . . . just in such a meadow, a wet meadow, ah, ah, ah. . . . He then embarked on another long story of the one other only flower, which was possibly the gardenia, ah, ah, when he was in Rome, so many years ago, he, the

august papa, had one a day, yes, to wear, a gardenia, it cost only about 30 Groschen, ah, ah. . . . If there could be ONE flower dearer to him than the narcissus, ah, it was the gardenia. . . . [Y]ou do seem to have a most dynamic way of busting into his unconscious.[63]

THE FOURTH MONTH

On May 1, H.D. had a run-in with armed soldiers on her way to the opera where she had gone despite Freud's warnings not to leave her hotel; she was interrogated and for this purpose had to pass the barbed wire behind the barricade. The Viennese were intimidated by this military show of force, and none of Freud's patients, except H.D., came for their appointment that day. Her venturing out to meet with Freud despite the danger in the streets proved something important, H.D. felt.

> The Professor said, "But why did you come? No one has come here today, no one." . . . I was the only one who had come from the outside; little Paula substantiated that when she peered so fearfully through the crack in the front door. Again, I was different. I had made a unique gesture, although actually I felt my coming was the merest courtesy. . . . I did not know what the Professor was thinking. He could not be thinking, I am an old man—*you do not think it worth your while to love me*. Or if he remembered having said that, this surely was the answer to it.[64]

H.D. continued to be upset about Freud's birthday and the upcoming move to Grinzing. The move was visible now, with stacks of cases and trunks lining the walls of the hallway. The consulting room and study, too, were affected by the turmoil, since Freud was taking along a number of books and art objects. Between these external events and the difficult work on her dream, H.D. was anxious and exhausted. She was looking forward to things settling down again.

In the meantime, she was still not sure what to do about the dog. She had made no commitment to Freud and begged Bryher, who was writing regularly to Freud and Anna, not to let him know about her conflict. She told him that her taking the dog to Switzerland depended in part on the puppy's health, to which Freud replied that since she was going to be in Vienna for another two and a half months, there would be enough time to see how it would develop. But this was the beginning of May, about five weeks before H.D.'s planned departure. In a letter to Bryher she comments about this mistake on Freud's part, wondering whether to contribute his statement to a simple confusion about the dates or whether he liked her so much he wanted her to stay longer.

On May 3, H.D. wrote Bryher triumphantly that Freud had spoken to her about a new theory, one he dared not write about for fear of making enemies of women. The theory concerned penis envy and included, in particular, the notion that it was a central ingredient in the development of all women, not just bisexual and homosexual women. What pleased H.D. even more than Freud's willingness to mention the new theory to her was the thought that she and Bryher might have had something to do with Freud's discovery:

> We have evidently done some fish-tail stirring, and if papa bursts out like the Phoenix with his greatest contribution NOW, I feel you and I will be in some way responsible. . . . [P]erhaps you and I . . . ARE to be instrumental in some way in feeding the light. Now you see all this in the unconscious may also be assisted by our liking the little dog. . . . [W]hile this idea of his is at work, and while I am on the operating table, I must, must, MUST feel that he has our sympathy about the doglet. It may date to the fact of his daughter dying with the trouble I had, in 1919. Papa was most concerned for my "pregnancy symptoms," and I think DOES link me up in some way with that daughter, who not only died like that but who also lost a child.[65]

To H.D.'s great relief, the Freud household finally moved to Grinzing in early May. Freud greeted her in the garden and after their appointment showed her around. H.D. liked it; in fact, she found the couch here more comfortable and was satisfied that Freud had brought enough of his art pieces to make the summer residence feel like home. Due to the general chaos resulting from the move, H.D. was able to meet other family members. She described her first visit to Bryher:

> He began bewailing how upset he was that he had no place here to wash after Yofi licked him. . . . Papa insisted on seeing me to the front door later, through the house. He hurled his magnetic hands skyward . . . saying, "My poor wife has had such a terrible time arranging all this." We got out to the front door . . . and there we caught "vif" two old ladies, obviously lady Sigmund and her sister. . . . I was so glad to add these to my collection. We also ran into a tall youth . . . the grandson. So now I have got a lot of the family on the map, due to the general confusion and everybody not knowing front door . . . from back. . . . It's terribly funny, and I am extremely glad for the change. I think it is good too for the unconscious.[66]

In her analytic sessions H.D. presented several dreams that clearly indicated her fear about the change of location.

May 6 was Freud's 77th birthday. Freud did not like birthday celebrations and did not cancel his patients. H.D. wrote to Bryher that his study was filled with flowers. But he himself, she thought,

> looked very wilted and sad. I don't think he likes to be reminded of his age. . . . I felt awful as papa looked so frail and I had no flowers. . . . He . . . said, "I do really thank you for not bringing me flowers." I think he meant it. He has probably spent the day making lovely speeches. I was so terribly upset about him. He was simply a thin silver edge of flame, and so tired.[67]

Freud confessed in the following hour that the birthday had been a "horror" to him and that seeing his patients had "kept him alive between callers."[68] As she left, he gave her a bouquet of orchids.

The confusion in the Freud household continued for a while, giving H.D. the opportunity to get to know everyone. The waiting room was part of the living room, and she could listen to Mrs. Freud's conversations with her neighbors and watch maids hurrying back and forth, dogs (there were now five) running in and out of the consulting room and up and down the couch, and Freud's grandchildren playing with the dogs. The chaos notwithstanding, H.D. was once again enjoying her analytic hours. In fact, she felt that the work was going better, and she had begun writing again. An event that importantly influenced her analysis at this time was the discovery of D.H. Lawrence's correspondence. Reading the letters had a profound impact on her and stirred up memories of the traumatic war years. While this was painful, H.D. was also aware that it would help her psychoanalysis. On one occasion, after she had played with Freud's grandson and dog, Freud told her that he was much concerned with the future of his grandchildren. H.D. felt that this was one of his main worries, and she asked Bryher to write him a note reassuring him that she would always look out for them.

The Lawrence letters were now becoming the focus of the analytic work, as H.D. told Bryher:

> I have been soaking in D.H.L. letters, not too good for me, but Freud seems to agree with me for once. Evidently I blocked the whole of the "period" and if I can skeleton in a volume about it, it will break the clutch. I only build up on the old foundation. . . . The "cure" will be, I fear me, writing that damn volume straight, as history, no frills . . . just a straight narrative. . . . I keep dreaming about literary men. . . . It is important as book means penis evidently and as a "writer" only am I an equal, in the right way, with men.[69]

When H.D. complained at this point about a painful toothache, Freud gave her the name of his dentist, warning her, however, "He is just one third your size."[70] Her fears surrounding this event were worked out in a dream.

The dogs continued to provide a lot of the entertainment, positive and negative. She described to Bryher how Freud had rushed to the rescue when Yofi attacked one of her puppies:

> We had been to the kitchen to see the pups. Freud ran like lightning and flung himself on the floor and pulled them apart, all his money fell out and Anna and the maid rushed in. . . . [A]nd there was Freud sitting on the floor with all his money rolling in all directions. . . . Very funny. And tragic . . . shows just how terribly young he is . . . a born fighter, so frail.[71]

Freud told H.D. that his wife found the dogs to be very disruptive and that she might associate them with her six children, all of whom she had had within eight years.

In the meantime, H.D. was trying to write a straight narrative account of the war years she had talked so much about to Freud. He encouraged her following through with this project and made it clear that he thought it would be important to write it from the point of view of a historian rather than that of a poet, that is, as objectively as possible. From her dreams, Freud told her, he could see that in her unconscious she had made a connection between these and other, earlier, experiences and that the analysis was now essentially over. One of the tasks remaining was the writing of that book.

Thoughts of death, although diminished, still haunted her. When Bryher mentioned to Freud in a letter that she was concerned about H.D.'s safety in Vienna, H.D. told her not to worry him.

> He was so vague and saint-like about it, and god knows he must be alarmed, and if he were actually attacked like that, you know, Fido, he might die, an old man of 77. . . . [I]t IS actual life and death to them and I dare not alarm them to this extent. . . . But Fido . . . Freud might easily die of the shock . . . he is burning in a thin flame now. It's sometimes terrible. . . . He is so old and god-like and frail, and I feel sometimes the psychoanalytic hours with outside people are all he gets of peace; he more or less told me so one day.[72]

Freud, at this point, was suffering from an attack of colitis but continued seeing his patients. H.D. realized that it immediately made him think of death, as he told her that she should get as much as possible out of psychoanalysis *now*. Seeing him in this physically weakened state—with a hot-water bottle to ease the pain and his women going in and out to administer medications—was frightening to her. H.D.

tried to convince him to rest for a few days, but he just shrugged it off. In fact, she got the impression that it was important for him to continue with the analytic hours, as though they kept him going: "If he lets go, I suppose he's afraid he will collapse."[73] She was worried that he might die; she told Bryher that she was glad about having started the analysis in March, when he was well. With the termination date now fast approaching, she began to make plans for the time after leaving Vienna. She thought about going to London and spoke with Freud about the possibility of continuing her psychoanalysis there. He recommended several analysts.

THE FINAL MONTH

It was the end of May. Up until this time H.D. had accepted that Bryher was pursuing a relationship of her own with Freud. But now when Bryher seemed to be getting too intimate with him, H.D. got angry. Bryher had mentioned someone's name in a letter to Freud without explaining who this person was, as though she assumed he should know. H.D. was furious about this and accused her of trying to interfere with her analysis.

> I spent half my hour yesterday telling Freud . . . who "Elizabeth" was. He was simply floored. Do be careful, when you write. Is it your unconscious that wants to believe he knows all about you . . . or do you want him breaking into my "hour" with questions about the whole menage. . . . Fido, you know you haven't been analyzed by him. He said the whole letter meant nothing though it was a specially charming one. He was most, most interested . . . most. But do remember, Fido, he has NOT analyzed you and call people by their names.[74]

With three more weeks left in the analysis, H.D. was once again feeling the strain of her work with Freud. She was still upset about his illness and found the work on the written account of her relationship with Lawrence and the war years difficult. The multiple interruptions of her sessions caused by the many dogs in the Freud household seemed particularly annoying, and she had not yet found a way of telling Freud that she was not going to take the puppy. During this time she had a dream that, she thought, finally completed the picture of her analysis. In this dream H.D., Bryher, and another woman are watching a play, written by a man, whose protagonist is cheating on his wife. This makes her think of penis envy, and she is amused. Out in the country they see the moon; it is larger than the sun and has all the colors of a rainbow. In it sits a beautifully dressed woman, an Artemis perhaps, or Virgin Mary. She is pregnant. A bird flies across the moon. Freud told H.D. that this dream conveyed an "almost perfect mythological state."[75]

Analyst and patient agreed that the dream—the three sisters and heavenly mother, the moon—was about homosexuality. The men were present only in a play, although they were symbolically transformed into the bird, or Holy Ghost, or "pregnancy agent," since the "band of sisters," of course, [could not] contemplate the 'father' as fertilizing element, in the pure state of homosexuality."[76] H.D. connected her fear of being moved, about which she had talked to Freud previously, with the fear of her homosexuality. After the dream she felt weak and tired, as though she had finally given birth. She also noticed that the pregnant woman in her dream was not phallic as earlier mother images had been. "[T]he phallic-mother," H.D. wrote Bryher, "was a layer before the final moon-mother. This was no phallic mother, the bird was phallus. So now I am in this pure spirit-mother state, and very happy . . . if I were not so weak. Just like having a pup, with pains too."[77] After this dream she felt that now the psychoanalysis was definitely over and that the remainder of the time would be spent merely with tying things up.

But it was not over yet. In these last couple of weeks of her analysis, H.D. found herself increasingly at odds with Freud's interpretations. She noticed that the writing of the book was getting easier—and that the more she liked it, the more she hated psychoanalysis. Freud told her that her dreams were expressive but that some link seemed to be missing. H.D. had her own ideas about what that was.

> I suppose it is the "father" vibration, for we can't, no matter how we idealize the mother-idea, get rid of the father. . . . I think I have made some funny pure classic transference, and that certain things, the "ball," these doves, represent "father," but do not link up with the actual personal father. I think the link is the star-stuff, but as S.F. once or twice has given such a snort when I have gone into star-states, it sort of cripples me.[78]

Astrology seemed to provide the link. It was in between astronomy, her father's science, which she had rejected, and the world of mysteries and magic to which she thought she belonged. And Freud, like her father, represented science and ultimately did not accept this aspect of her individuality. Here they had come to a point of real disagreement. H.D. thought about talking to Freud about this.

> And that is where, in a way, S.F. and I part company. I suppose that, too, is symbolical of my leaving my own home and its surroundings and the strictly, so-called "scientific." But I think you will agree that

star-fish stuff is my real world. . . . S.F. may nip it in the bud tomorrow. But I don't think he will. I think I must simply have it straight out with him. He is good, you know, too good, and he has to stick to his scientific guns, but I have to stick to mine too.[79]

H.D. left Vienna on June 15, 1933, and joined Bryher and Perdita in Kenwin, a house in the foothills of the Swiss Alps, built by Bryher. The possibility that she might return to Freud at some point in the future was left open. For a while she was able to work on her writing, but she soon began to feel increasingly alienated from her friends. In the following summer she suffered another breakdown. She believed it was precipitated by the news that one of Freud's patients, J. J. van der Leeuw, the theosophist from South Africa whom Freud respected a great deal, had died in a plane crash. Van der Leeuw had preceded her on the couch, and she sometimes saw him leave on the way to her own hour. It was van der Leeuw who had wanted to exchange treatment hours one day and to whom Freud had introduced her on the Grinzing lawn so they could work it out.

A YEAR AND A HALF LATER

H.D. returned to Freud and resumed her psychoanalytic sessions on October 29, 1934, for one more month. Freud was now 78. She said that she had come to tell him she was sorry about van der Leeuw's death: "I said to the Professor . . . 'I felt that you and your work and the future of your work were especially bequeathed to him. . . . I know that you have felt this very deeply. I came back to Vienna to tell you how sorry I am.' The Professor said, 'You have come to take his place.' "[80]

Again H.D. stayed in Vienna by herself. Freud told her after several appointments that he could sense a powerful resistance or fear in her that he was anxious to analyze. Being back with Freud made H.D. feel better immediately. In a letter dated November 2, she told Bryher that she was already making great progress and that this time the psychoanalysis was less intellectual and funnier. She was also writing again after having difficulties doing so in the preceding few months; it appears that she was still working on the book she had started in Vienna the year before. Her disagreement with Freud over the importance of astrology continued. She still felt that she was right, but she was more accepting of their differences. Overall, she was less preoccupied with the analysis between treatment hours than she had been the previous time. She brought in dreams for almost every appointment and noticed that they were frequently about beautiful nude women. They were the key, she thought, to the present work. But it was not all easy and comfortable. After one week she wrote Bryher, "Papa is drilling away like mad, this time. . . . I am simply shattered each time."[81]

H.D. saw Freud five times a week during this period. The fee was slightly higher than it had been the time before. As before, Freud did not like the idea of Bryher paying the full amount in advance for fear that he might not be able to finish the work. It had been arranged beforehand that H.D. would stay for a particular number of sessions, amounting to about five weeks, which she felt would be sufficient to get through her crisis. At the heart of it, she and Freud agreed, was the fear of death she had experienced in Kenwin. Freud thought that it probably stood for an earlier, suppressed fear that her father would die. She had later repressed the memories of her brother's and father's deaths, and was conscious only of her anxiety about war and atrocities, which in terms of the political realities of the time seemed justified. Freud made the link between her fear of death and their relationship:

> Papa thinks that I am now afraid he will die, which is of course a regular psychoanalytic proceeding, but it is a very real thing, as mixed up with my own terror of crossing streets, etc. So I think, I AM NOT so happy this time—it is *reality*, rather than "dope," it is doing the trick. . . . It is again raining, rather agonizing as streets are slippery and my phobias grow on me.[82]

From a dream Freud gathered that Bryher's paying for the analysis had contributed to H.D.'s resistance. In the dream H.D. is riding a black horse. Suddenly, the one horse turns into two—or it becomes a horse with two heads—pulling her into opposite directions. After a tremendous struggle she is finally able to get through a forest, and the horse becomes one again. She takes it to a place near the town where she was born and has tea with her old nurse or aunt. She gives the woman a tip, against her protestations, saying that half is for her and half is for the horse. It embarrassed H.D. to have Freud point out the connection with the fee: She had left all the financial arrangements to Bryher. She told Bryher about his interpretation:

> Freud thinks I have been worried in unconscious about your paying my bills here, or about his asking more this time. All this is terribly awkward for me, for I did not know I was paying "less" last time. I think there has been some conflict in *his* mind, as you were so terribly meticulous last time and I broke into my own psychoanalytic time, two or three times, to ask him for the bill. He said you had sent money after psychoanalysis was over, that more than "made up." But I didn't know there was anything to "make up" for.[83]

Perhaps H.D. did not want to know about the details of Bryher's financial transactions with Freud. Freud's insistence on discussing this matter now made her wonder, as previous comments had, whether *he* had some kind of complex about it. In a letter the next day she wrote that perhaps Freud was trying to "sting" her about the money. A little later she found the conflict worked out in a dream that related to her brother in some fashion.

Even though Freud knew that H.D. was planning to stay for approximately four weeks, a termination date had not been set explicitly. H.D. was wavering as to whether she should extend her visit for an extra week or so but essentially did not want to go beyond the time agreed upon initially. Freud told her that it was up to her, that he could arrange to see her for longer, and that there was no rush about the decision. At this point, two weeks into this analysis, H.D. felt they had understood what was at the root of her most recent crisis—her fear of death. But a different part of her history came now into focus. "I have had every nerve in my whole tail exposed by papa in this psychoanalysis," she wrote Bryher. "The whole now of psychoanalysis is about death, not so very cheerful, but I suppose the boil in the unconscious has bust. Apparently it is terror, ALL the time, in the unconscious of the old group."[84] "The old group" is a reference to some people Cecil Gray, her daughter's father, was involved with two years after Perdita's birth, when H.D. approached him about child support. The group included Gray's friends Butts and Heseltine and had formed around an Aleister Crowley, who allegedly belonged to some kind of satanic cult. There were tales of drugs and extortion, people being driven to suicide, and so forth. Freud found this matter significant and pursued it with interest.

> Papa seemed surprised that I hadn't mentioned the "Butts" world before. It apparently is very important to him—represents the "father who terrifies" . . . and is probably the clue. It made all the Corfu experience, I think, click into shape for him. He was very kind before but thought my ideas of psychic phenomena a little extreme, I know. Now he seems to see how it works.[85]

H.D. was not actually involved with this group, but the rumors she heard about it terrified her. She was afraid of becoming a blackmail victim herself; in fact, she had always had a fear of some secret being found out about her. Freud reinterpreted this as a "father-terror complex" and connected it with her identification with various other victims—for example, van der Leeuw and people she had known who had committed suicide.[86] Being victimized meant death. Furthermore, H.D. had experienced Freud as a blackmailing father in connection with the discussion about money.

Papa is most kind and helpful since I had linked him up with
blackmailing father-symbol. . . . [I]t came out, about the fees of
psychoanalysis. Papa is very clever. He said it was "father" this time,
and evidently I linked it up with the usual textbook, Zoo primal scene.
If it is the case, you will see that the weeks here have been of immense
benefit.[87]

In a dream, H.D.'s ex-husband, Aldington, is in bed with Bryher, to
whom he is married. He shoots first her and then himself. This dream was
clearly based on the story of a friend, Conrad Aiken, whom H.D. had
tried to get into analysis with Freud. She had mentioned him to Freud,
but he merely said that nobody could be forced to get help. It was Aiken's
father who had killed his wife and then himself. H.D. thought that the
dream was an elaboration of the primal scene: The father kills the mother
in bed. Once again, she noticed the importance of the victim theme. Her
mother in the dream was a victim, as H.D. feared she herself might
become. Bryher stood for the mother, but H.D. realized that she could be
the father, too. Freud thought the dream was perfect in its symbolism.
H.D. went on now to reinterpret the Van Eck saga: He stood for the father
from whom she wanted a son, except that a sexual relationship with him
would have meant death, physically as well as socially. She wrote Bryher
about some further associations:

My child is a golden child Christ-child off the X mas tree, all very clear
at the age of seven. But child meant primal scene, meant being "killed"
by a man, the father. . . . [M]y father gives me, the Virgin, at the age
of 7, a son. Or SUN. There seems to be no special fight or rivalry with
my own mother. I am simply a wonderkind with a divine child, "born
in Bethlehem."[88]

The dream also emphasized the way in which H.D. felt she had lost both
her parents and explained how all her subsequent love relationships were
based on this mixture of love and terror. Freud told H.D. that he thought
her fondness for things magical was really just a different kind of poetry,
a suggestion H.D. rejected. She wrote Bryher that she did not simply
accept everything Freud said anymore but that she was now able to argue
and disagree with him. Freud, she thought, seemed to have become
friendlier after they discovered the origin of her fear.

Since Bryher had already paid Freud a certain amount of money for
the analysis, H.D. now, toward the second half of November, asked him
to find out how much time was left. Freud promised to ask his son Martin,
who was managing his financial affairs. Martin reported back that enough
money remained for about nine more sessions. This meant that H.D.
would leave Vienna on December 2, as originally planned. In the course

of her conversation with Freud over the length of her stay, she gained the impression that he did not want her to leave. Still nervous in the wake of their recent conflict about money, she now tried to handle this matter in as business-like a manner as possible.

When they started the second round of their work together, Freud had been persistent in confronting the fear or barrier he perceived in H.D.'s free associations. The probing quality of his questioning had felt like "drilling" to her, but now that her victim complex had come into focus, his attitude changed and he seemed more affectionate. She also learned something new about his technique.

> I told Freud a long tale yesterday, full of important details. When I had used up the hour he said, "I can tell from the way you speak, that you are hiding things. So I did not have to listen. You ran your articles together. You did not speak clearly." . . . Evidently papa simply listens to the wave-lengths. But . . . he was right, as we are on early masturbation layer.[89]

In the same letter to Bryher just quoted, H.D. passed on a piece of gossip about Freud that delighted her in that it suggested the possibility of sexual escapades on his part. She heard that he used to be accompanied on some long journeys by his sister-in-law Minna while his wife stayed home with their little children.

Evidently in relation to his observation earlier that she was hiding things, Freud now gave H.D. an interpretation that concerned her sexual identity as well as her writing difficulties. She wrote to Bryher, "He said, 'You had two things to hide, one that you were a girl, the other that you were a boy.' It appears I am that all-but extinct phenomena, the perfect bi-. . . . [I]t seems the conflict consists partly that what I write commits me—to one sex, or the other, I no longer HIDE."[90] H.D. could well connect this interpretation with her experience of discomfort about being a woman: It made her feel trapped. She agreed that she seemed to be switching back and forth between being a woman socially and sexually and being a man in her writing. It was perhaps an old theme—being rejected by her mother for her brother, not being the son her father wished her to be, and so forth—but it had never seemed quite this clear and she felt grateful that Freud had made it explicit.

Bryher had apparently been trying to make a donation to the Sachs Fund and now decided to give the lump sum to the Vienna Psychoanalytic Society. The advantage of this to the Vienna group was that they could collect the interest. Freud was very pleased.

> Then he went on purring and wanted all the low-down on the English group, and I told him how they wanted to get you and your dollars into

the London set, and how you wouldn't. . . . [T]he purring nearly shook the house down, like an old lion whose heart's desire has been fulfilled. I could hardly get on with psychoanalysis. . . . I am so very happy this came about before I left. It makes such a dramatic finale.[91]

In later letters H.D. made a couple of references to this donation, telling Bryher that it motivated Freud to tell her the truth about the terrible fate of the puppy they never took, and that he seemed to consider the gift a symbol, "The gold, the Frankincense and the Myrrh touch."[92]

Freud told H.D. that her dreams and associations had become so clear there was no need for him to talk at all. He had agreed with her that the earlier dream of Aldington shooting Bryher in bed was a representation of the primal scene and that all the later traumas she had discussed with Freud had their foundation in that image. She had lost both parents, which resulted in her bisexuality, signifying loss and independence at the same time. Being bisexual meant being man and woman simultaneously, as well as neither, and it meant being perfect. Writing provided an opportunity to obtain the perfect balance. Freud now considered H.D.'s psychoanalysis finished.

Before her last appointment, H.D. brought a plant to Mrs. Freud as a farewell present. She left it with the maid and went to the waiting room, but Mrs. Freud followed her, thanked her effusively, and left.

> Papa appeared, said nothing of mama, but solemnly presented me with one of the orange branches with leaves and oranges, all terribly symbolical. Well—I just managed to get through my hour, but had a very weepy time when I got back. I must say I am in love with the old mama, too. . . . So I think you may rest assured that I am well fixated and, probably, for life on the famille Freud.[93]

H.D. told Bryher that she was very happy about the results of the psychoanalysis but that it would be a while before they would fully take effect.

Freud's Analysis of Joseph Wortis

J OSEPH Wortis was born in Brooklyn, New York, on October 2, 1906. He attended New York University and then studied abroad; he graduated from Vienna Medical College in 1932 and interned at Bellevue Hospital in New York City. After his internship the young doctor, sponsored by Havelock Ellis, the English physician and eminent sexologist, and by Adolf Meyer, the leading American psychobiologist, returned to Vienna on a fellowship, which he used to support his analysis with Freud. Wortis was 28 when this analysis began; Freud was 78.

Following his analysis, Wortis returned to the United States and joined the staff of Bellevue Hospital in 1935, where he was the first to undertake the electroconvulsive shock therapy of severely disturbed patients. During the next several years he held faculty appointments in psychiatry at Johns Hopkins, Columbia, and New York Universities. During World War II, Wortis served in the Public Health Service and attained the rank of lieutenant commander. Following the war, he directed the Division of Pediatric Psychiatry at Jewish Hospital of Brooklyn and later became professor of psychiatry at the State University of New York at Stony Brook. Throughout his career Wortis was an active researcher in neuropsychiatry. He died in 1995 at the age of 88. All of the quotes in the following treatment narrative are from his book *Fragments of an Analysis with Freud* (1984), unless otherwise noted.

It seems apparent in Wortis's case that the patient entered treatment with what we might call a character transference, or what Freud described to Wortis as a "character resistance." Symbolically, the treatment quickly took on the aspect of a wrestling match whose instinctual sources and meanings the patient defended himself against through intellectualization and acting out. Certainly, analyst and analysand were immediately contentious, descended to unseemly bitching at their lowest points, and often enough nipped, whined, and barked their way through the treatment hours—with Freud's chow, Yofi, present as an interested, but more restrained, spectator.

* * *

NEGOTIATIONS

The first meeting between Freud and Wortis lasted 15 minutes. The young doctor had requested an appointment shortly after his arrival in Vienna in the beginning of September 1934. He wanted to discuss his work and, in particular, his plan to study psychoanalysis. Freud was again spending the summer in Grinzing. Wortis arrived for his appointment a few minutes early. A maid told him to wait; Freud was very punctual, she said. After the previous patient left, Wortis was shown to the consulting room, where Freud welcomed him with a handshake. Wortis wrote, "He was short of stature, slight of build, and looked intensely pale and serious. His manner was direct and to the point, and he wasted no time on ceremony. It fell upon me to explain my presence."[1] As Wortis was fluent in German, the analysis was conducted in German.

Wortis told Freud that he had received a fellowship to research the nature of homosexuality. Havelock Ellis and Adolph Meyer, who were overseeing the project, had offered him the position the previous year, but Wortis at that time was just finishing his psychiatric internship and had accepted only on the condition that he first have time to acquire a more general knowledge of psychiatry. An agreement was reached, and Wortis went to London to visit several clinics and consult with experts. He now wanted to further his knowledge of psychoanalysis, which he thought would be helpful from a theoretical and clinical point of view. When Wortis was finished with his account, Freud concluded, "Sie wollen also Psychoanalyse lernen [So you want to learn psychoanalysis]."[2] Freud's words made Wortis uneasy; they were clear and decisive, while his own feelings about psychoanalysis were quite mixed. Earlier in the year he had written to Meyer:

> Though I am myself skeptical of the dogmas and claims of the psychoanalysts, don't you think it would be worth-while to learn something of the subject at first hand? . . . I think that it is of first

importance too to acquire the techniques I may need later, since the
book-learning and clinical experience will come easier then. I mean
some training in physiology, in biochemical endocrinology and in
histo-pathology, as well as in psychoanalysis (or something similar).[3]

But, for now, he did not make mention of these thoughts. Freud told him
that the only way to learn about psychoanalysis was to be analyzed. There
were good analysts who were relatively less expensive, he said, but if
Wortis could afford his fee, perhaps with the help of the fellowship money,
he would consider doing the analysis himself. Wortis was impressed with
Freud's straightforward manner.

Freud sat opposite me with a little table between us, facing me directly.
Sometimes he bent sideways and leaned on his desk, looking keen and
mousy. His speech was low and muffled and the metal appliance in his
mouth . . . seemed to cause him much annoyance. His German was
precise and deliberate, and he spoke his syllables and words with
emphasis. He made no bones about asking me a number of questions
about myself: my age, my experience, was I neurotic, was I sexually
abnormal, was my wife with me now? If I was no . . . severe neurotic—
an analysis would not be a matter of more than a year, but then . . . I
would naturally learn a lot.[4]

Before he left, Wortis mentioned hearing that Freud's health was precari-
ous. Freud dismissed his concern. The meeting was over.
    Havelock Ellis, who not only was involved with the fellowship but
also was a mentor to the young Wortis, had offered to help further his
chances with Freud by sending a letter of recommendation. He made it
clear, however, that he was strongly against Wortis undergoing a didactic
analysis. Should Wortis go ahead with the plan, Ellis, who had grown
increasingly distant from psychoanalysis, advised that he make sure to
keep his independence from psychoanalytic doctrine and follow Freud's
example of scientific research rather than his teachings: "If you are
psychoanalysed you either become a Freudian or you don't. If you don't,
you remain pretty much where you are now; if you do—you are done
for!—unless you break away, like Jung or Adler or Rank."[5] But Wortis
was not to be dissuaded, and Ellis wrote the promised letter. Shortly
thereafter Ellis received this response from Freud: "To me a talented
pupil is naturally preferable to a patient. I would be glad to take him on,
provided a certain condition is met, and provided I remain well enough
to work. The condition concerns the honorarium. I am unfortunately
not so successful that I can disregard the matter of making a living, but
must sell my few hours of work dearly."[6] If it could not be worked out,

Freud added, he would refer him to a distinguished student, perhaps his daughter Anna.

Meyer, in contrast to Ellis, supported Wortis's plan and helped procure the necessary funds. By the end of September the negotiations were settled. On October 1, Wortis and Freud had another meeting. Wortis made a point of noting in his journal that he himself was late. "This time I kept Freud waiting, for I came a minute late, and noticed him standing at the window looking out to the gate when I passed through. . . . Freud waved me to a chair and I again talked first."[7]

Wortis announced that $1,600 had been made available for his analysis. Freud quickly calculated that the sum would last four months, which he thought was a reasonable amount of time, particularly since Wortis was a student and not a neurotic.[8] In a training analysis, completion was less imperative, Freud said, so he should consider their work an introduction to psychoanalysis; he might someday want to pursue it further. But, wrote Wortis, Freud was not willing "to use this limited sum of money to give me mere informal theoretical instruction, such as Ellis suggested and I desired."[9] Perhaps, suggested Freud, Wortis wanted to consider being analyzed by his daughter; the money would last longer. But Wortis's decision was made.

> I replied it was simply a question of Freud or nothing for the present; so far as I was concerned I was ready to start, on the understanding that these four months would be reasonably adequate. Freud thought this possible, but it would depend on my . . . receptive capacity, and my . . . supply of neurotic material, which after all every civilized person has. . . . I accepted the proposal.[10]

Wortis spoke of Ellis's disapproval of his being analyzed and read parts of the Ellis letter described above. Freud concluded that Ellis had turned against psychoanalysis. Many people, he said, could accept it only in a limited way. Wortis thought Freud's attitude toward his critics rather arrogant. He warned Freud that in the end he himself might reject psychoanalysis, and he found Freud's suggestion that doing so would constitute illness on his part "disagreeable."[11]

Freud doubted that Wortis, at 28, would be competent to form an "independent judgment."[12] Wortis replied that he might discover something entirely new, something even Freud had overlooked. He reminded Freud of having belittled his critics by writing that those who had not been analyzed were in no position to judge psychoanalysis because they did not know enough and the criticisms of someone who had been analyzed were suspect because they might be caused by resistance. And what about the fact that Freud himself had never been analyzed? Freud answered:

> "But I discovered analysis. . . . That is enough to excuse me." . . . For the rest, he could interpret his own dreams and recollections. I need have no fear, he went on, that I would lose my independence; and that, he added, is a lesson: when I come to analyze others I will discover that my patients will have exactly the same feeling. . . . "We shall see."[13]

Freud reiterated, perhaps now wishfully, what he had said to Ellis, namely, that he much preferred a student over a neurotic patient.

THE FIRST WEEK

Shortly after this meeting Freud wrote Wortis that he could see him for his first appointment on October 9, 1934. Wortis was to confirm the proposed date by phone but chose to write a note instead. The time was good, he told Freud, but it was really his sponsors who had to finally approve their arrangement. After all, they were the ones paying for it. He did not foresee any problems since the $1,600 had already been authorized. But should there be some obstacle, Freud would be paid for services rendered. When he arrived for his appointment, Freud let him know what he thought of this contingency plan.

> Freud had me sit down and made it clear that he was displeased with this uncertainty: I either agree or disagree to start, and he was unwilling to start before the financial matter was settled. I said that was only a matter of a few days, until my last week's letter arrived in the U.S.A. . . . I did not feel it was worth this long discussion; I had no secret plans, and felt there would be no difficulty at all. "But," said Freud with a characteristic turn of phrase, "the fact remains that you wrote this letter. You didn't want to take the responsibility on yourself, you wanted to share it with me."[14]

Freud eventually agreed to begin under the condition that Wortis request final approval by telegram.

Freud then explained the ground rules of psychoanalytic treatment. The patient and doctor should meet five times a week, for one hour per meeting. It was advisable, he said, to allow two weeks before deciding whether an analysis was workable. He took Wortis to the couch, had him lie down, and sat behind him in a chair. The couch, he continued, was important so the patient could relax and, moreover, he himself did not like being looked at all the time. Furthermore, it was imperative that Wortis speak his mind as freely as possible; psychoanalysis required a measure of honesty that was not usual in regular social contact. Of course, everything he said would be kept private unless the material was of scientific interest and could contribute to the development of psycho-analytic theory. He asked Wortis about his knowledge of psychoanalysis, which turned out to be negligible.

> He found it most convenient, then, he said, to assume I knew nothing, though I was not to take offense, since it was a mere matter of convenience. I remember saying I was first attracted to Freud through Max Eastman's book, *The Sense of Humor.* "A bad book!" said Freud. "And now," he went on, "you can start and say what you like."[15]

Wortis began by talking about the one time in his life when he had had what resembled neurotic symptoms; but, he was quick to add, they had since vanished. The episode occurred during his psychiatric intern-ship at Bellevue the year before. He had felt alienated from his environ-ment and friends, listless, and self-critical. He had difficulty working, was unable to keep up with his studies, doubted his intellectual abilities, and developed somatic symptoms. The feelings persisted for a while even though he knew that they had no basis in reality. It so happened that at this very time he was offered the fellowship, which quickly improved his mood and restored his self-confidence. By the end of the analytic hour, Wortis felt uneasy: he did not like thinking about painful things and was worried that they might distract him from other pursuits. But even more disturbing was this:

> There was the unpleasant prospect of developing what Freud called *Widerstand,* or resistance, against him, my present lord and master; who sat in quiet judgment while I talked, like a stern Old Testament Jehovah, and who seemed to take no special pains to act with hospi-tality or reassurance, but had instead needlessly disturbed our friendly association by what seemed to me to be an over-emphasis on money matters.[16]

Wortis was angry that Freud wanted him to send the telegram and complied only grudgingly. The next day Wortis announced that his resistance now amounted to 17 schillings and 29 groschen, the price of the cable. Freud smiled and said he understood. He asked when an answer could be expected, and he then reminded Wortis where he had left off the day before. Wortis spoke of his relationship with Ellis and provided further details about his background and relationships. Among other things he mentioned that he had met his wife at a young age; they had been separated for several years while he was studying abroad, which had created some difficulty. Freud said, "There is an element of dependence in every relationship, even with a dog."[17] Freud's chow was sleeping next to the couch. When speaking of Ellis, Wortis praised his flexibility and tolerance for other people's points of view.

This second appointment was more to the young analysand's liking; none of the topics he discussed upset him. Freud did not say much.

> He seemed to be a bit hard of hearing, but did not admit it. On the contrary he continually criticized me for not talking clearly and loudly enough. "You're always mumbling," he said with some petulance, and he gave a mumbling imitation, "like the Americans do. I believe it is an expression of the general American laxity in social intercourse, and it is sometimes used as . . . *Widerstand*."[18]

Wortis replied that it was, in his case, only a matter of habit and promised that he would try to improve his enunciation. He then questioned whether free association was truly possible. The content of his thoughts, he argued, would necessarily reflect the context, namely, Freud and his theory of sex and neuroses. Freud told him to continue saying what was on his mind.

In the third hour Wortis was not sure of what to say. Freud repeated that he should speak his mind. Still nothing in particular occurred to him, so Wortis decided to present his ideas about psychology. He thought that neuroses could be prevented by making changes in the person's environment, since neuroses were the result of a conflict between the individual and the external world. Freud remarked that prevention was not up to the analyst, but Wortis insisted that nothing would stop *him* from doing so if he wished. He believed also that physical well-being and an active, productive life were essential to psychological health. Too much emphasis, in his view, was given to intrapsychic problems. Freud just said, "It is not so simple," but otherwise refrained from commenting.[19] Wortis eventually returned to speaking about his personal life.

> I proceeded to give an account of my vicissitudes in love and life. Freud made friendly and sympathetic remarks here and there, seemed to think I was well-trained in honesty, and said it was "*eine gute Vorbereitung für die Analyse* (a good preparation for analysis)." I said I was not overmuch interested in myself, and felt better when I simply went about my work. "That is of interest, too," said Freud. "You have made everything you said up to now so clear it has not interested me either."[20]

Wortis left the hour unsure of how to take Freud's comment.

Freud told him the next day that he should talk more about his problems. Wortis first denied that he had any, saying that the depression of the previous year was gone and that he had remembered it only because he was in psychoanalysis. But then he mentioned having a schizophrenic relative, which worried him now that he had learned that heredity might be a factor in the etiology of psychiatric illness. Freud argued that the heredity in schizophrenia was recessive, but Wortis disagreed. Then he attempted to discuss other troubles. "I proposed to talk this hour of all the various painful thoughts I had ever had . . . various conscience-pangs, self-reproaches and anxieties, though none of them seemed any longer of any real consequence. I didn't know whether Freud grew more interested. I tried hard to think of real problems I had had."[21]

THE SECOND WEEK

A week after they started meeting, Freud moved from his summer residence back to Vienna. Wortis was feeling well and energetic and continued with the presentation of his history. At one point he reminded Freud of a comment he had made a couple of sessions before:

> I made some reference to his earlier remark that my account was uninteresting. Freud explained that he had not meant he was uninterested, but that he thought *I* was, because I kept speaking of clear, superficial things. I explained that it was not exactly uninteresting to me, but that generally I found I was not very content when I was overconcerned with myself and that I might also have a certain amount of apprehension about the course the analysis would take and what unpleasantness it would reveal.[22]

Freud listened but did not say much. Wortis mentioned in passing that, at the suggestion of Ellis, he might visit with Stekel.

The following day, Wortis returned to the subject of schizophrenia. He quoted another author whose point of view was identical to his own, namely, that schizophrenia was "not a disease entity but a symptom complex of a group of diseases with some common features."[23] Freud was annoyed. His voice was sharp when he replied that the etiology was not well understood and that, moreover, it was not a symptom but a syndrome. Then he said:

> "I have noticed, during your recitation up to now, a special characteristic: a tendency to leave the solid ground of facts, and to talk in a general way of things that are not intelligible to me. You talk away, for example, of your feelings and experiences without so much as telling me where and when they all occurred. Furthermore, I have been able

to observe in you a tendency to lose yourself in abstractions and to talk of things of which you have no knowledge, in a way which reminds me of someone whom I know, Havelock Ellis. He speaks freely of things about which he has no knowledge at all without so much as concerning himself with the literature. How a man with any knowledge of things could ever have recommended you to Stekel . . . is beyond my comprehension."[24]

Freud now told Wortis in no uncertain terms what he thought of his one-time follower.[25] Wortis was taken aback, but reassured himself with the thought that this had nothing to do with him. Nevertheless, he apologized for some of the things he had said but added that, after all, he was just speaking his mind and Freud ought to expect that not all of it would make sense. He then repeated his thoughts about schizophrenia, sounding less dogmatic this time. Freud listened attentively and encouraged him to keep associating. Wortis continued with his history. When he concluded that he had had a very happy childhood, Freud said, "I am very glad to hear that . . . for it is certainly unusual."[26]

Wortis began the following hour by talking about politics but soon returned to Freud's criticism of him. He objected to being thought a bad scientist and said that he was not going to give it much attention. Freud replied that he had merely observed "a certain undesirable *tendency*."[27] At least, Wortis continued, he was not the only one suffering from this affliction: Freud had accused Ellis of the same shortcoming. He spent the rest of the hour with further details about his childhood and first sexual experiences.

Approximately 10 days after they had started the analysis, Wortis had completed the account of his history and brought in his first dream. His impression that Freud had been waiting for him to do this was confirmed when Freud said:

> "There are people who cannot be analyzed, often perfectly normal people . . . and I have been waiting up to now to see if you would tell me of your dreams, because that is how we shall now proceed with the analysis. . . . The next few days will show whether enough material for an analysis will be forthcoming."[28]

Freud did not think that this dream, in which Wortis was kissing Freud's maid, was significant.

Wortis returned the following day with another dream: He is visiting Ellis and his wife, Françoise. Françoise has forgotten his name, and then appears to want to kiss him. There are so many other guests and servants that Wortis worries the house might burst. Ellis's hair was recently cut; Wortis wondered whether it would be long and shaggy. Suddenly there is fog. Ellis explains that this is a natural phenomenon. The dream suggested to Wortis, among other things, that he wished Ellis were more conventional and accepted in higher levels of society. Freud agreed with parts of his interpretation but added that "other things were hidden from [Wortis] because of [his] preconceived scientific opinions or prejudices. The dream was an anxiety dream, and since the only abnormal thing that had come up was the hypochondriacal idea, it was concerned with that." Freud then said that Wortis's "future instruction would have the purpose of removing [his] scientific prejudices."[29]

Wortis recalled another dream in which he is lying in bed while a cat licks and chews at his little finger. The only association that occurred to him was that the dream was a response to an actual event during the night, that perhaps his finger had gotten caught somewhere. Freud reminded him that he had refuted such explanations a long time ago. He concluded that the two last dreams could not be interpreted entirely, because Wortis's scientific prejudices acted as resistance. Wortis asked Freud whether the analyst was supposed to be as honest as the patient. Freud answered that the analyst must use tact and not lie. Wortis then wanted to know whether Freud would tell a patient that he was a hopeless case.

> "You mean, do I think you are neurotic," he said. I laughed, and said I didn't think I meant that; I didn't consider myself neurotic and didn't think I would be. At the worst, I was concerned to know whether Freud considered me neurotic, but I had not intended to ask him. I continued to talk freely.[30]

Wortis reminded Freud of his earlier comment that it was unlikely that his depressive symptoms had just disappeared. He himself did not believe that a recurrence was likely. Also, was a doctor not supposed to reassure his patients? Freud repeated that if his "little phobia," as he called Wortis's reaction at the time, was not analyzed, it would very possibly return.[31] Wortis left the hour in good spirits; if Freud thought of his symptoms as a "little phobia," not much could be wrong with him.

The next day Wortis felt somewhat ill, a fact he attributed to work-related difficulties and being run-down physically. Freud suggested that perhaps it had to do with the analysis. But Wortis minimized the impact of the suggestion by remembering Freud's words from the day before. Having a little phobia, he said, did not seem like such a bad thing; moreover, he still was not convinced he had ever had one. It was true, he admitted, he had a tendency to criticize himself and worry about his abilities, but it was no more serious than that. Freud replied that it was normal for young people to doubt themselves and that the question of whether or not he had a phobia was not important in and of itself. He himself used to have several phobias; they were common but warranted exploration. Wortis then inquired whether he could ask general questions occasionally. He wanted to know, for instance, what Freud thought of the role played by constitution in the etiology of homosexuality. Freud answered that it seemed an important factor. At times, Wortis acknowledged, he had worried about his masculinity. Freud, who was more talkative in this hour, reassured him: "Nobody is completely masculine."[32] Wortis then mentioned that one of the things that used to bother him about himself was his high-pitched voice, a characteristic he shared with Ellis; he attributed it to the tightening of muscles in the vocal chords, a result of tension. When Freud seemed skeptical, Wortis insisted.

> It is at least true as far as I am concerned. . . . "Don't say things that way," said Freud; "it makes a bad impression." I apologized, and said I simply meant that the observation held good for me, though maybe not for others. "And this brings us to the dream you had," said Freud, "for I have observed certain feminine elements in it—which by no means implies that you are effeminate," he added. He then said, "The analyst does not say all that he thinks, but lets the subject talk until he reaches a point or topic that can be used in the analysis."[33]

Freud proceeded to interpret Wortis's dreams from this angle. For instance, he said, the servants entering the house were symbolic of a womb giving birth to children, and Ellis and Françoise stood for his parents. His avoidance of Françoise, who was trying to kiss him, was a denial of his wish to kiss her. The cat sucking his finger in the third dream represented a child feeding at the breast. Wortis agreed only with the observation that Françoise's wish to kiss him was a disguised oedipal wish. The rest of the interpretations, he told Freud, seemed "far-fetched." He also rejected the idea that the dream about Ellis and Françoise was an anxiety dream. Freud reminded him, "We are simply working with suppositions, since the analysis has only just begun."[34] However, he dismissed Wortis's theory that dreams were merely a way of justifying the subject's moods and warned him that his theoretical ideas would not hold up once he began working on his dreams.

Toward the end of the hour Wortis mentioned that he and his wife, who was 28, were considering having a child. Freud seemed surprised that they were still undecided and commented that they ought to have children while his wife was still young. Wortis replied, "I shall tell her that . . . I know she'll be very glad to hear that Professor Freud thinks so."[35] Freud shrugged off the sarcasm and just added that it made sense from a medical point of view. The subject of Stekel came up again. Freud asked Wortis to tell Ellis in his next letter that "he really should be ashamed of himself . . . that he recommended Stekel to [him] in any sense whatsoever."[36]

THE THIRD WEEK

After two weeks of analysis, Wortis was not happy. He tried, quite consciously, to get off the subject of his own internal life by turning to more general topics. He talked about Hirschfeld, who Freud thought was "scientifically dumb."[37] When Wortis commented that Hirschfeld seemed to be homosexual, Freud replied:

> "He doesn't *seem* to be . . . he *is*, and he makes no secret of it. And not only is he homosexual, but he is perverted in other ways. I have heard from a patient of mine that he satisfies himself in the most perverted way." This was said with emphasis, almost as if in moral indignation, and I did not know how it accorded with Freud's views on the analyst's discretion.[38]

Wortis asked Freud's opinion on whether monogamy would survive in a socialist society. Freud pointed out that he seemed to expect psychoanalysis to have ready-made answers for everything; this was not the case. They spoke of Russia. After talking about his own relationships and insisting that he had come to accept monogamy, Wortis mentioned a dream from the previous night in which two black people were fighting each other and one was killed. His only association was that he had heard news of a possible revolution. A further dream from the same night, one with sexual content, also yielded little by way of associations.

> I said in the course of the discussion of the dream that I preferred a "common sense" psychology. Freud then said I had too many ideas and too few associations. Either I could not relax myself sufficiently or else I had tremendous resistance. . . . I did however discuss various memories and details, and Freud said in conclusion, "We have moved a little forward."[39]

During this time Wortis was attending lectures in neurology, which quite fascinated him. He told Freud the next day that the organic basis of mental functioning was what he would study if he had the choice. Freud responded, with an edge in his voice, that Wortis might indeed be better suited for that than psychoanalysis. Hearing this did not please Wortis; maybe he should consider changing direction professionally, he said. Freud replied, "A person who professes to believe in common sense psychology and who thinks psychoanalysis is 'far-fetched' can certainly have no understanding of it, for it is common sense which produces all the ills we have to cure."[40]

Wortis defended himself by saying that he had not meant to be critical of Freud's ideas when he called his interpretation of the dream "far-fetched." As to the common sense psychology, he added, he just wanted a psychology to be simple. Freud responded that the more simple it was, the greater the likelihood that it was wrong. But changing direction now, he continued, or terminating the analysis was not called for. There were things to learn. Wortis challenged Freud's comment that he would be better suited for neurology: How did he know? Maybe he would not be good at anything? Freud replied that some people were better suited for certain professions than others and that from experience he could judge a person's talent for psychoanalysis. Wortis was furious:

> "That is too bad . . . since I shall probably continue my work in psychology anyway. I consider you the greatest psychologist we have had, and I should have liked nothing better than a word of encouragement from you. I'm sorry I have gotten just the opposite." "There is no need to show *you* any consideration," said Freud. "You have a degree of self-confidence that fortifies you against criticism. It is really enviable."[41]

Wortis said that Ellis, in contrast to Freud, had been supportive of his professional pursuits.

> "Ellis's interest in you was just part of his general kindness," [Freud replied.] . . . "Don't you think Ellis has any talent for psychology, either?" I asked. "He certainly hasn't," said Freud.[42]

Wortis did not agree that he had a lot of self-confidence. Ellis had told him once that he lacked it. He was mollified a little when Freud conceded that he seemed basically a happy person and that some measure of doubt was normal. He told Freud that he regretted the fact that they were having differences and that his theoretical preconceptions were getting in the way. He wanted to change this. Then he told Freud a dream: He is climbing up a ladder to get a book for a female doctor, while a Professor Marburg is standing by. The dream was about his wish to help Freud with something he could not do because of his age, Wortis thought. But Freud suggested a different interpretation:

> [He] finally concluded that the ladder meant coitus, the books meant women, and the woman in the background was my wife. I was showing the old Professor, in short, how well I could practice coitus, to the

annoyance of my wife. "That sounds at least plausible," he concluded, and I agreed. When I shook hands to leave I said again I hoped he would change his opinion of me in time and would tell me when he did, so that I could repress the memory of what he said today. "No need for that," he said.[43]

The next hour Wortis resumed where they had left off the day before. He was still fuming over Freud's comments and said to him: "Self-complacency and lack of talent are a bad combination . . . and I don't feel flattered."[44] Freud replied that such a combination of attributes was rather common, but then added that he had not come to a final opinion about Wortis's personality. This did not reassure Wortis. He complained that Freud's way of dealing with his resistance was unscientific and ineffective.

> Freud agreed. "It's true," he said, "that the young analysts analyze too much. But I was using the method in private, in the course of an analysis, to remove *Widerstand,* though it was appropriate just the same." "But you simply increase the *Widerstand* by such methods," I said. "That would just be a personal *Widerstand,*" said Freud, "and would be easy to dispose of."[45]

Wortis then told several dreams, the themes of which involved feelings of failure and impotence. But Freud was still interested in a dream from the day before that had to do with a teacher, guilt over missing school, and certain numbers. After Wortis had associated to the possible connection between the numbers and money, "Freud hit the sofa and said, 'I have an idea! But I don't know whether it will please you. Or rather I don't care whether it pleases you; I don't know whether it is appropriate to the dream.' "[46] His idea was that Wortis had a fantasy of missing some analytic appointments so that he could keep for himself the money that belonged to Freud. Wortis rejected this interpretation, but Freud took the opportunity to tell him that he would have to pay for every appointment whether or not he made use of it. Notwithstanding Wortis's protest, Freud asked whether there was any reason, from a financial point of view, to believe the analysis might have to end soon. No, there was not, Wortis replied. Freud seemed less angry.

In the following hour Wortis spoke about neurology, the conditioned reflex, and other related topics. When Freud did not respond, he told him another dream, which brought him back to the recent argument. He criticized Freud for being intolerant of people who disagreed with him:

> "You act as if psychoanalysis stood high and perfect, and only our own faults keep us from accepting it; it does not seem to occur to you that

it is simply polite to reckon with one's own prejudices too." "An analysis is not a place for polite exchanges," said Freud. "I observed that you had a certain amount of *Widerstand* and set about to remove it." "I can't see the technical advantage of that," I said, "for my pleasure in analysis is certainly diminished." "It is best to leave matters of technique to me," said Freud.[47]

Wortis also complained that Freud had tried to devalue his relationship with Ellis. He felt that Freud took him seriously but thought that he "sometimes took offense at the wrong things."[48] Wortis let slip that he was talking to his wife about the analysis; she had begun to add her observations to what was going on. Freud was not pleased. He told Wortis, "The analysis is a private matter between you and me, and you ought not to speak to anyone about it. You want to learn more about human nature . . . because you are ignorant and I am here to teach you. An analysis is not a chivalrous affair between two equals."[49] Even though Freud seemed, overall, more friendly, Wortis was depressed when he left the hour.

Freud invited Wortis to read any of his books despite having thought initially that it would get in the way of the analysis. Wortis took advantage of the offer and complimented Freud in the following session on some of his papers. He also apologized for his defiant and arrogant attitude. "Conceit is an unpleasant quality," he told Freud. "I don't like it in others, and I am sure they don't like it in me. I should be perfectly willing if you treat it as a bad symptom and cure it if you can."[50] He added that he felt hurt at the thought that Freud did not like him. When Freud explained that his comments were not meant to reflect his personal opinion, Wortis was relieved. He related some dreams that showed his concern over losing Freud's love and then returned to the subject of his phobia. But neither he nor Freud had changed their position on this question. Wortis was disappointed.

THE FOURTH WEEK

In the next couple of hours, Wortis initiated discussions of various topics he found interesting. They all underlined his tendency to explain psychological matters on physiological grounds. He asked a number of questions, such as what the difference was between a neurosis and normal difficulties and whether homosexuality was pathological. Freud answered his questions until he got annoyed when Wortis pointed out that he had not written about the role of financial difficulties in the formation of the neuroses:

"I don't understand how you can concern yourself with such purely conventional problems . . . what is a neurosis and what is not a neurosis, what is pathological or not pathological—all mere words— fights about words. First learn something about neuroses and then you will know what a neurosis is. With all your scientific curiosity . . . there are big loopholes in your interests. Your business is to learn something about yourself. You talk of this and that, about money and abstract questions, because you are not really interested in yourself—you have no curiosity."[51]

Freud repeated that Wortis had too many prejudices, as reflected in his wish for a "common sense psychology," his calling psychoanalytic inter- pretations "far-fetched," his attempt to explain psychological matters through conditioned reflexes, and his suggestion that one ought to "let sleeping dogs lie."[52] He thought Wortis's idea that psychoanalysis could create a neurosis was preposterous. It was possible that Wortis was not neurotic, Freud continued, but his symptoms deserved exploration. But Wortis was obviously reluctant to do that, he said, and was only justifying his fears on theoretical grounds. Wortis agreed.

"That is quite possible," I said. "I am perhaps afraid of my unconscious." "Of course," said Freud, "that is why you make all these difficulties. I tell you, it may be just as well if we make this our last hour"—he had given me the month's bill at the outset—"if you feel that way about it." I said I would be sorry if the analysis had to stop. I would do what I could to cooperate and would always be ready to change my views. "All right," said Freud, "but you ought to be ashamed of yourself for acting that way, grumbling and growling for three days because I said this or that to you. You will have to give up your sensitivity. You ought to understand that I am not interested in passing judgment on you. If I say anything it is only for the sake of the analysis."[53]

Wortis tried to explain his challenging attitude by emphasizing the limited amount of time he was going to have with Freud; he wanted to learn as much as possible. No, Freud answered, Wortis was trying to impress him; furthermore, he continued, arguing over words was not what psychoanalysis was about. Wortis replied that, after all, Freud was a genius and finding out what he was thinking was very inspiring. He promised again to change his attitude, and he returned to the subject of his difficulties from the previous year.

In the dreams he reported the following day, Wortis continued to criticize Freud. In one he implicitly reproaches him with being bourgeois. Adolph Meyer is in the dream, and Wortis remembered his insecurity before meeting him. Freud concluded from Wortis's associations that his

obsessive ideas were connected to his love relationships. Wortis replied
that he could not quite accept the interpretation; Freud answered, "You
just mean you don't like it."[54] In the next hour Wortis complained that
he had found out not only that he was neurotic but also that he had
compulsive ideas and that they were not just a thing of the past but
current in his life now. Freud repeated that a neurosis from the past could
well recur during an analysis. He thought Wortis's response to his observations remarkable.

> "[T]he interesting thing is how you turn everything into a judgment
> on you, as if that were the only thing that mattered." "I don't like to
> lower my opinion of myself, without getting something in return," I
> said. "That is not a scientific attitude," said Freud. "You have not yet
> completed the transition from the pleasure principle to the reality
> principle."[55]

The rest of the hour was unproductive. Wortis could not think of
anything to speak of except scientific matters, which Freud said was only
a manifestation of his resistance. At the end of the hour Wortis took care
of some financial business.

> I paid Freud for the month and asked him if he would receipt the bill
> with the conventional German phrase, "*dankend solviert*"—"received
> with thanks"—so I could send it to America. "Why with thanks?" he
> said. "I give you something which is at least as valuable as what you
> give me." "I thought it was a mere technical formula," I said. "Among
> businessmen, maybe," said Freud.[56]

It was now almost a month since Wortis had begun his analysis. He
was not pleased with the way things were going. He spoke again of his
symptoms from the year before, repeating that he thought they were
normal considering the circumstances; in his opinion, Freud exaggerated
their significance: "Mountains were being made out of molehills."[57] Freud
agreed that the neurotic mechanisms evident in them did not mean that
he was seriously pathological. Wortis expressed his gratitude toward Ellis,
who had been so helpful then, and he praised other attributes in his
mentor's character, such as respect, tolerance, consideration for others,
and shyness. How helpful Ellis's kindness ultimately was, Freud replied,
remained to be seen. Wortis protested that it was comparable to the
importance of the positive transference in psychoanalysis.

> "No," said Freud, "I am glad you brought the question up, because I
> can clear up the misunderstanding: the positive transference is not part
> of the psychoanalytic therapy. The psychoanalytic cure consists in

bringing unconscious material to consciousness; to this end the positive transference is used, but only as a means to an end, not for its own sake."[58]

Freud then spoke of Ellis's criticisms of psychoanalysis, which he thought showed only that he understood nothing of the subject. Wortis defended Ellis feebly. At the end of the hour he asked Freud to read a paper he had written, an assignment from the hospital where he was receiving his psychiatric training. Freud said it was not a good idea.

THE SECOND MONTH

In the next couple of hours Wortis presented some short dreams. In one of them a woman dies during an operation. Wortis wondered whether it was his wife but then rejected the idea. Freud insisted that his first association could be trusted and asked him what came to mind about the numbers in the dream, namely, 3 schillings and 65 groschen. When Wortis could make nothing of them, Freud suggested that they might be a reference to the number of days in the year. Among other things, this made Wortis think of how long it would take to cure his neurosis, but he quickly added that this was probably quite irrelevant to the dream. Freud complimented him for having worked better that day.

In another dream Wortis's landlord accuses him of being a criminal. In his treatment hour Wortis recalled that Freud had commented earlier that it was of no consequence to the analyst whether the patient was a saint or a criminal. Wortis had been offended by this remark, convinced that Freud really thought he belonged to the latter category. Not getting a response, he turned his attention first to the dreams from the day before and then to his current studies of the brain and its relation to the sexual functions. Freud, who seemed distracted and spoke little during this hour, asked whether he was hoping to find the cause of homosexuality there. No, Wortis replied, but he ought to be familiar with it because of its significance for sexuality. He was enjoying his work and was pleased that his symptoms from the year before had disappeared. Freud remained skeptical. It now occurred to Wortis that he had not acknowledged the homosexual content in two previous dreams. "I think I revived these denials with mischievous intent, and proceeded to talk of some homosexual acquaintances, and of my thoughts on homosexuality. Freud listened. I said I was glad I was not homosexual and felt perfectly satisfied with heterosexuality."[59]

For the second time in four days, Wortis was late for his appointment. He insisted that there were good reasons for the delay, but Freud interpreted it as resistance. There was less tension in this hour; thoughts on anti-Semitism and England provided some common ground. When Wortis could think of nothing else to say, Freud reminded him:

> "Just let your mind drift. . . . You don't have to speak of things that happen now. . . . Anything will do, past or present, since it is all of one piece, and our purpose is to see the structure of your mind, like an anatomist." I spoke of various little things, such as peculiarities I thought I had. I said for example that I sometimes absent-mindedly scratched my head or cleaned my nails; "You ought to break yourself of the habit," said Freud.[60]

It was now five weeks since the analysis began. Wortis asked whether there was a difference between a regular and a training analysis. Freud answered:

> Only insofar as the material and progress of the analysis is different. With a neurotic patient the analysis must follow the fluctuations of symptoms and *Widerstand* and adapts itself to the state of the patient at any given time. With a healthy student, these fluctuations don't always occur unless he is neurotic to start with or becomes neurotic during the analysis. I have been waiting for this question, for I knew that you would pretty soon ask where we were getting, and I must admit that from an analytic point of view we are not getting far. You are a so-called normal person. . . . The only reason you have for cooperating in an analysis is scientific curiosity. You notice my methods with you have changed. I tried to use personal criticisms for a while, but you were too sensitive to it, and began to criticize me in turn, so that I have had to treat you more carefully.[61]

Now that Freud had said he was essentially a normal person, Wortis began to argue about *that*. He sometimes had long spells of sadness, he said, although not as of late. Other people, he continued, might also disagree with Freud's positive impression of him, and he enumerated several criticisms that had been leveled against him. With Ellis he often felt self-conscious, wondering what Ellis would think of him if he knew how mean he could be. Perhaps he had difficulty accepting success, but he sometimes wished that people would admire him less and like him more. In fact, a certain amount of failure might be good for him and inspire humility. Freud reminded him that he had not much liked hearing criticisms. Wortis defended his reaction and then talked more about his inadequacies. Before long he returned to the subject of the difficult two months of the year before. Freud pointed out that he had not been able to make any observations about his behavior without Wortis exaggerating their meaning. Yofi prevented a repeat of the old argument. At this point Freud's big chow was heard scratching on the door, and Freud rose, as he often had before, to let the dog in. Yofi settled on the carpet and began licking her genitals. Freud did not approve of this behavior, and tried to make her stop. He said, "It's just like psychoanalysis."[62]

It was now the middle of November. Wortis was late for his treatment hour again and promptly met with Freud's interpretation that his behavior indicated resistance. He added, "Work well now to make up for it."[63] Wortis spoke of a dream: He is asked to evaluate the mental state of a girl who is brought in by her parents, only to realize that the father, who seems very irritable, is suffering from an incipient general paresis. Wortis thought the father in the dream was himself; he could be irritable. He also remembered saying to his wife the night before that Freud did not think he was neurotic; he had added jokingly that Freud had been fooled since he was actually quite crazy. Freud quickly set things straight and said that

> he did not mean to flatter me by calling me healthy. I was just one of those supposedly healthy . . . people who went about without much trouble because their complexies were stored away out of reach. "There is no reason to feel proud of it," he said. "One likes to be healthy," I said, "but I was not altogether sure you did me justice."[64]

Wortis admitted that Freud's statement about his obsessive tendencies had worried him for fear it might be true, but he now began to argue whether his preoccupation could actually be considered obsessive. Freud commented that it made no difference what he said because Wortis always found a reason to disagree. Wortis disagreed with this, too, and then talked again about the less attractive aspects of his personality.

> "Sometimes I think I may antagonize people on purpose. Maybe I like to fight too much." I talked on and on this way, and seemed to reach low depths. Afterwards I felt I had drawn a much less favorable picture of my relations to my group than I deserved. Freud made little comment. I felt baffled again. At the end of the hour I shook hands with him. "I hope I develop a neurosis," I said in all sincerity, meaning, I suppose, that some interesting neurotic material would emerge.[65]

After five weeks in treatment, Wortis had to admit that something was the matter with the analysis. It was not advancing. Freud emphatically agreed with him, saying that he did not understand what was wrong. He suggested that they give it another two weeks and that if things did not change for the better, they end it. Wortis felt he was to blame. He reiterated his desire to learn about psychoanalysis and its technique and felt puzzled as to what was getting in the way. Was he just healthy? Even so, he said, it was odd that the analysis was revealing nothing. On the surface it appeared that everything was simple, even his dreams, Freud observed. He thought that Wortis had "character resistance."[66] Wortis did not like the idea of interrupting the treatment, but his criticisms of himself for being so obstinate did not convince Freud.

> I said I had moods of self-reproach for being so resistant a subject during analysis. "Character resistance" suggested something undesirable to me, and I was sorry I was so difficult. It is true, Freud replied, that I was critical of myself and thought frequently of myself, as an intelligent conscientious person should do, but it was all superficial; in my unconscious I was proud and complacent, and resistant to the analytic procedure in spite of my avowed respect for Freud. "A person is made up of several parts," he explained: in some respects I felt inferior perhaps, but not in others, and my professions of respect were just the familiar counterpart . . . to my real feelings.[67]

Wortis repeated his regret over being so difficult. By the end of the hour he was depressed.

In spite of Wortis's protestations that he wanted to change his attitude, the stalemate in the analysis continued. On the surface he tried to comply with the demands of the treatment but then, without fail, found opportunities to argue about some theoretical problem. In the dream-work he insisted on his concrete, physiologically based point of view, which Freud countered with deep interpretations. In one hour Wortis presented a dream that involved his wife and a fish-chopping machine. Freud exclaimed, "That's what I call a real dream," and proceeded to interpret the fish as a penis symbol.[68] His subsequent short lecture on dream analysis did not convince Wortis.

> I . . . left in some distress, because I did not believe in this psychoanalytic theory of dream symbols. Although I recognized the partial truth of many of Freud's observations it still seemed to me that he neglected the fact that the thinking process in dreams was basically affected by the *inefficiency* of mental functions under the conditions of sleep.[69]

He continued to feel out of sorts for the next several treatment hours. In one dream Wortis watches a man performing sword tricks on the stage of a theater. The man is dressed in military apparel. Suddenly, looking down into the orchestra, Wortis becomes aware that the man could fall and calls to his wife for help. The patient's only association to the dream concerned a newspaper article he had just read that discussed the possibility of war and mentioned the opening of a play on the subject. Freud suggested that the dream was concerned with the primal scene, with the sword standing for penis and doing tricks with it standing for sexual intercourse; the military angle represented the aggression that children often associate with sex. He explained the symbolism of falling by way of etymology: It stood for the feminine aspect and implied, from a linguistic point of view, birth or giving birth. In summary, Freud concluded, in the dream Wortis was watching a couple have sex and was bothered, in particular, because he identified himself with the woman. He reassured Wortis, who wondered about the homosexual aspect, that this was a dream typical of heterosexual men who were worried about their femininity. Wortis did not believe that he had ever seen sexual intercourse. In the following hour he mentioned that Freud's ideas about the symbolism of falling could be supported by statistics. Freud was annoyed. "That is a typical American idea," he said, "you can't study psychology with statistics."[70]

Wortis dreamed he had cancer of the face, from which he feared he might die. Thinking that he was now trying harder to comply with the principles of psychoanalytic theory, he suggested that perhaps the dream expressed his feeling that the analysis was making him ill. But Freud said it was a simple death wish: Wortis wanted him to die from his cancer (Freud had had cancer of the palate since 1923). Hearing this did not help Wortis's somber mood. In the next several hours he initiated more theoretical arguments about various aspects of psychoanalysis, all the while flaunting his agreement with Ellis's ideas. For a while Freud patiently explained the basis of psychoanalytic theory, but lost his composure once more.

> He then proceeded to criticize me roundly again for launching out into abstractions, though I defended myself with some confidence, for I did not believe that dreams are essentially different from other mental activity. "You ought to listen and learn," he said. "You have been receptive to Ellis, now you ought to learn something from me. I can't make a psychoanalyst of you in this short time, but I can give you the stimulus in that direction."[71]

Much to Freud's annoyance, Wortis kept holding up Ellis as the exemplary scientist. At one point, for instance, Wortis said: "Ellis once told me . . . that the older he got the less sure he grew of everything. I am curious to know if you have the same feeling."

> "I am older than Ellis," said Freud with emphasis, "and I can say that the older I get the more sure I grow of everything. . . . I have always criticized him for having made too few decisions. . . . And now in his

old age it is no wonder that he feels uncertain. You have the same fault, and you gave yourself away at the beginning of the analysis, by saying you were satisfied to be shrouded in the luminous mist of truth."[72]

THE THIRD MONTH

Wortis's criticisms of psychoanalytic theory did not let up. At one point he interpreted a dream with sexual content from the point of view of homosexuality, a ploy that he knew was "mischievous, though psychoanalytically proper."[73] When Freud rejected the interpretation, Wortis gleefully noted that he had found a way to make Freud talk: He only had to contradict him. It supported his conviction that Freud was essentially negative and pessimistic by nature, a trait he thought was reflected in his theories as well. But his triumph over being able to provoke Freud did not make up for his dissatisfaction with the analysis:

> My mood at this time began to be a combination of scientific bewilderment, because I could not accept many of Freud's conclusions and was essentially out of sympathy with his attitude, and personal displeasure, for I did not like the idea of being constantly probed for morbid features of my psychology.[74]

It was now the middle of December. Wortis kept arguing, Freud kept trying to convince him of the validity of psychoanalytic ideas. Freud found his patient's resistance to the work with dreams especially trying. The following is a typical example of an argument over a dream interpretation: In the dream a detective shoots Wortis in the shoulder after his refusal to stop walking. Wortis offered this interpretation: "I am threatened, and told unpleasant things during analysis, but I don't care and go my own way."

> Freud grew indignant: "An attitude of that sort makes further analysis impossible: it is purely emotional." "Naturally," I said, "it is emotional; rationally nothing ought to bother me. I don't see why that need interfere with the analysis." "What about the wound and the bandage? Why were you shot in the shoulder?" "I had to be shot somewhere; why not in the shoulder?" I said. "Perhaps I was lying on my shoulder, or had my hand on my wife's shoulder during sleep. . . . I don't know if that is significant." "Everything is," said Freud. . . . Freud was irritated.[75]

Wortis did not follow the rule of free association, which Freud continued to point out. Among other things, Wortis attacked psychoanalysis on grounds that it was too bourgeois and insisted that he could not accept the concept of sublimation and its good for civilization. Freud was talkative and patient and tried to explain what he was missing in his arguments. Apropos of a discussion about the merits of a society regulated by the government versus one in which free enterprise was encouraged, Freud ended the hour with an anecdote: A Jew in the army was intelligent but lazy; his superiors finally recommended that he buy a cannon and go into business for himself. Freud chuckled, but Wortis was not amused.

Through his outside studies Wortis now became familiar with the newly discovered insulin shock treatment for schizophrenia. He was impressed with this method not only for its own sake but also because it gave him further ammunition against Freud in that it seemed to confirm the organic basis of this illness. Freud emphatically opposed this viewpoint and said that psychoanalysis had never been able to cure organic cases. Wortis replied that in the United States a lot of money had been wasted by doctors who had tried psychoanalysis as a treatment for diseases that were of organic origin. But Freud was not impressed: " 'What your American *crooks*'—Freud used the English word—'do is certainly not representative or typical of the science of psychoanalysis.' "[76] Wortis reminded him of a paper in which Freud actually acknowledged that the therapeutic gains of psychoanalysis were limited to the mild neuroses. He then reported a dream—which he thought disproved Freud's theory of wish fulfillment—in which insulin treatment fails as a therapeutic measure.

> "This is the opposite of what I really wish," I said, "and seems to refute the theory of wish-fulfillment in dreams." Freud argued back energetically again. "It does nothing of the sort," he said. "That is one of the apparent negatives of wishes which I have already explained and settled long ago." "That was probably in your book on dreams, which I haven't read for years," I said. "You probably have never read it," said Freud, but added, "If you have read it, you haven't understood it."[77]

Wortis did not accept Freud's interpretation of his dream, namely, that his real wish was for Freud's method to fail.

In discussing another dream, Wortis found occasion to say that he thought Freud was not treating him very nicely. He added that he knew he had something to do with this and would try not to generalize from his behavior toward him. In response, Freud repeated what he had said before, that is, that his only purpose was to teach him something about psychoanalysis. Wortis admitted that he did not quite understand why Freud was keeping him if he found him so difficult; he had been half-expecting Freud to terminate the analysis. The main reason he was doing that, Freud replied, was that he did not like giving up on something once he had started. He chided Wortis again for being so argumentative. Wortis answered that he was just speaking his mind.

> "What am I to do then?" I asked, "not tell you what I feel?" "Accept things that are told you, consider them, and digest them. That is the only way to learn. It is a question of . . . take it or leave it. The trouble with a . . . didactic analysis . . . is that it is difficult to give convincing demonstrations, because there are no symptoms to guide you." "Why am I such a difficult subject?" "I told you once before, it is your narcissism, your unwillingness to accept facts that are unpleasant."[78]

The next day Wortis was in good spirits and reported two dreams that, as he himself suggested, showed his narcissism. When Freud agreed with the interpretation, Wortis, dismayed, became silent; he then resumed his criticism of Freud for being so intolerant. Before long his thoughts returned to the subject of his narcissism. He reminded Freud of having once called his self-confidence enviable; now he was finding fault with it. Was that not a contradiction? As for himself, he said, he could not see the advantage of being self-critical and morose. Furthermore, it disturbed him to be considered part of the group of dissidents or opponents about whom Freud had made such scathing comments. Freud asked him to identify these individuals.

> There was Stekel, for instance, I suggested. "You called him such names that I was terrified; and there was Hirschfeld, whom you called perverse and obnoxious." . . . Freud objected to this and said he had said nothing of the kind (he had), that I did not remember what he said, and that it would be very painful to him if I repeated anything of the sort to anybody.[79]

The following day Wortis was still busy refuting the idea that he was narcissistic. "My 'narcissism' did not seem to be a general phenomenon: I stood in real awe of Ellis, for example, and trembled in his presence."[80] Moreover, Wortis said, Freud himself had not seemed particularly self-effacing when he was young. Meanwhile, Ellis, in his letters, supported and even encouraged Wortis's challenging attitude.

In the beginning of January, Freud reminded Wortis, who was spending much time discussing the insulin shock treatment, that with only one month left he should not distract himself so much from his analysis. He chided him again for being so resistant.

> "Here we are moving to the end of the analysis, and you still haven't grasped the fundamentals." I said I expected to study later and perhaps learn more when I did my own analyzing. "But you have no right to

analyze," said Freud emphatically. "You know nothing about it—you are just a *bloody beginner*." . . . "But I cannot, unfortunately, study forever," I said. "I have a research fellowship and have to do some research of my own. What will I live on otherwise!" "I recognize all that but it has nothing to do with analysis. You have a right to live, but not as an analyst."[81]

Freud was not done: He told Wortis that just *because* he was intelligent but ignorant about psychoanalysis he could cause much harm and that his efforts to teach him had so far been to no avail because of his arrogance and unwillingness to admit that he understood nothing of the subject.

When Wortis protested that Freud might have discouraged him with his outspokenness, Freud replied:

> "I don't think I could have done you any harm. Either you are so conceited that my remarks don't bother you, and you run me down in return, so that I have another enemy—which doesn't matter—or else you take notice of what I say, and act accordingly."[82]

Wortis had learned nothing from him, he continued; he did not even believe in something as fundamental as the theory of wish fulfillment in dreams. Wortis then spoke of a dream in which he chose Adler over Freud. He had been present recently at a social event at Adler's daughter's house, and he now credited Adler with the social perspective in Freud's theory of homosexuality. Freud responded at length with a lecture concerning the position of psychoanalysis on social issues. At the end of the hour Wortis said that he would feel greatly honored if he could translate one of Freud's works. They had all been translated, Freud replied, and there would be no new ones. In the next couple of sessions Wortis spent much time discussing theoretical questions and brought in more dreams. Freud, who had been kindly and patient, eventually lost his temper again.

> This was one of the very worst. . . . I was again subjected to one of Freud's regular rough criticisms. The occasion was a dream which, I remarked rather facetiously, I was glad to say seemed quite normal. Freud made some sharp critical rejoinder, and I defended myself by saying nobody likes to hear of bad or morbid traits. Freud thereupon told me to give up my narcissistic attitude and be more receptive to what was said. "I am not so sure I am so narcissistic," I said; "I usually don't hesitate to recite my faults and weaknesses to others." "The reason for that of course," said Freud, "is well known: you tell other people, so that they may not tell you."[83]

Wortis was upset and felt humiliated; he spoke of his anger the next day. Freud, much friendlier again, encouraged him to express his feelings and listened to his complaints with "admirable patience."[84] He repeated that his remarks were not directed at Wortis personally.

THE FINAL MONTH

During the final month of the analysis, Freud complimented Wortis occasionally and offered him a copy of a book that had been difficult to find. In the middle of January the topic was, once again, Wortis's reluctance to accept psychoanalytic principles. Freud said he thought it was based on an unscientific attitude, namely, his unwillingness to deal with unpleasant truths. Wortis asked for examples. Freud reminded him of a particular dream.

> "In analysis," Freud warned me, "one learns what real conviction means, and I think there is reason to suspect that you are still not altogether convinced." "Because," I interrupted, "I was too proud to present you with an apparently contradictory dream?" "Fine!" said Freud with enthusiasm. "That's what I call real analysis." "Well," I said, "I hope I will learn in time." "That was fine!" said Freud again.[85]

For the next week Wortis engaged Freud in the discussion of a variety of topics, most of them not directly related to his analysis. Then, with only a week left, he suggested that perhaps he ought to review what had occurred between them.

> I had heard more bad things about myself than good, and my spirits were perhaps dampened, but on the whole it looked as if I would leave the analysis as healthy as when I took it up. "But you still have time for the funeral oration . . . " said Freud. "We have another seven hours or so, and plenty can happen by then; all this simply shows that you are anxious to get it over with." "Or else," I suggested, "I want to give you a chance to put in a few good words for me before it is over." "That is not my business," said Freud. "I told you unpleasant things about yourself to show you how honest one is in analysis."[86]

Wortis expressed the hope that Freud's criticisms did not mean that he was somehow worse off than most people. Freud repeated that he had seen no signs of a serious neurosis and that his rather mild symptoms did not take away from the fact that he was essentially healthy. Indeed, Freud continued, a neurotic tendency could be very motivating, particularly to a psychologist. He added that Ellis, for instance, must be sexually abnormal in some way. Wortis was so upset about this remark that he could hardly listen for the rest of the hour.

Wortis spoke of several dreams. In one he tries to get a friend and a woman doctor interested in him by talking about Freud; rather than saying that Freud has a fine intelligence, which is his intention, he says that he is in fine condition. Wortis attributed this to paraphrasia in dreams, a phenomenon mentioned by Kraepelin. Freud replied that the paper by Kraepelin was nonsense. It was silly to think, he added, that organic factors were involved here; it was simply a slip of the tongue, the meaning of which could be understood when analyzed. Freud was annoyed, a state Wortis inferred from Freud's tapping with his fingers on the top part of the couch. In another dream Wortis is late for a class and does his best to avoid the teacher's attention. The feeling in the dream reminded him of his reaction to Freud's comment about Ellis; he thought it was unfounded and devaluing. But Freud defended his hypothesis that Ellis was sexually immature by pointing out that he had a homosexual wife, no children, and was probably impotent, as evidenced by his inability to make decisions. Wortis countered:

> I insisted I never said his wife was homosexual. . . . He had no children because his wife was diabetic—besides, he was too poor; and as for the last argument, it was weak. Shakespeare made few judgments too—he saw too many sides to an argument. Freud was angrier than I had ever seen him. He sputtered: "Do you know Shakespeare, then, as well as you know Ellis? Anyway, he was a poet, not a scientist." Besides, what did I mean by now denying that his wife was homosexual?[87]

To contradict Freud's contention that Ellis might be impotent, Wortis reminded him of a poem by Ellis, which was in one of the books in Freud's waiting room. Freud asked him to get it, but did not think it proved anything. The argument continued the next day, but Freud was in a better mood and took back some of his statements, saying that they had apparently been based on false evidence.[88] However, he chided Wortis for his tendency to say things in their discussions that were not entirely accurate.

In the penultimate hour Wortis summarized what he had learned about himself in the analysis. He enumerated various things Freud had said about his inadequacies and personality traits. Freud made only occasional comments; he put his earlier statements in context and emphasized their objective nature. Concerning Freud's remarks about his patient's personality, Wortis wrote in his journal: "This was merely a description of my character type and ought not to be overestimated; it was a narcissistic attitude which he could not explain."[89] Wortis had countered by arguing that despite Freud's having found "distasteful elements" in his dreams, they were on the whole strongly normal. "Too strong in fact," Freud had noted.[90]

Analyst and patient met for a last session on January 31, 1935. Wortis mentioned that he had run into Stekel and conveyed some of the complimentary remarks Stekel had made about Freud. Freud thought they were inspired by nothing but arrogance and manipulation and talked about the discord between various members of the psychoanalytic group. In a dream from the night before, Wortis says good-bye to Freud and then tells a grandson of Freud's, who wants to study medicine and psychoanalysis, that the family name is a guarantee of success. The primary feeling in the dream was guilt, which Wortis attributed to his sense that he had failed in the analysis. Even though he had to hear a number of unpleasant things about himself, he said, he was pleased to have had the opportunity of working with Freud. He was going to consider what Freud had said about him and felt he had learned enough about psychoanalysis to be convinced of its scientific merits. He then mentioned that in the dream he asks Freud for a photograph; Freud immediately offered him one of his books instead, since he had no photos. Summarizing further what had occurred in their work together, Wortis said that Freud's ideas about socialism had been an inspiration. After spending the remainder of the hour talking about this topic, patient and analyst parted with friendly words.

CHAPTER FIVE

Freud's Analysis
of John Dorsey

J OHN Dorsey was born in Clinton, Iowa, on November 19, 1900, to Edward and Anna (née Looney). He received both his B.A. and M.D. degrees from the University of Iowa. In 1926 Dorsey married Mary Carson, with whom he had two sons, John Jr. and Edward. From 1930 to 1935 he was an assistant, then an associate professor of psychiatry at the University of Michigan. Following this he began his analysis with Freud and entered into a two-year course of postdoctoral study at the University of Vienna and the Viennese Psychoanalytic Institute. From 1946 to 1961 Dorsey was professor and chairman of the psychiatry department at Wayne State University in Detroit. Over the course of a long, productive career, Dorsey published numerous articles and books on psychiatry, including a biographical study of Thomas Jefferson and his own autobiography (Dorsey, 1980), written toward the end of his life. He was a president of the Michigan Society of Neurology and Psychiatry and the Michigan Association for Psychoanalysis. Dorsey died on August 6, 1978, at the age of 77. He began his analysis with Freud when he was about to turn 35; Freud was 79. All of the following quotes are from Dorsey's book *An American Psychiatrist in Vienna, 1935–1937, and His Sigmund Freud,* unless otherwise indicated.

Like Wortis, Dorsey seems to have begun his treatment with Freud with a character transference, but his was of a very different and more agreeable sort, namely, the idealizing paternal transference of the lovable baby of the family. "More agreeable" does not mean innocuous, however; in fact, this sort of transference presents the clinician with constant temptation—to which the naive, the greedy, and the unscrupulous can readily succumb. Indeed, Freud seems to have regarded Dorsey as an essentially likable and innocent American aborigine, one who was perhaps exasperating at times in his strenuous efforts to please him and gain his admiration. It is unclear whether Dorsey's overzealousness and tendency toward intellectualization were off-putting to Freud or whether Freud simply found him less interesting than other patients. In any event, Freud does not appear as engaged in this treatment as he does in the other cases. With Dorsey, Freud remains in the background and limits himself to encouraging the patient to free-associate.

* * *

John Dorsey arrived in Zurich at the end of September 1935. He was on an 18-month sabbatical from the University of Michigan State Psychopathic Hospital, where he had been first assistant director for seven years. Dorsey was visiting European clinics and hospitals to increase his knowledge of psychiatry and psychoanalysis.

Shortly after his arrival in Zurich, Dorsey began looking for an analyst. He interviewed both Oscar Pfister and Emil Overholzer, neither of whom was quite to his liking. Having no other referrals, he asked the advice of J. Michaels, a friend from the University of Michigan who was in analysis with Edward Bibring in Vienna. Michaels recommended that Dorsey try to see Freud and offered to contact his daughter Anna, through whom all such arrangements were made. In the middle of October, Michaels informed his friend that there was indeed a good possibility that Freud would analyze him. Dorsey wrote in his journal,

> I am vastly pleased to learn that Professor Freud is considering favorably my wish to do my analytic work with him. I am told that there is no difference between an ordinary and a training analysis, except that in the latter the training analyst must be qualified. All along I have stressed my *academic* interest in my analysis. I am elated, highly, over my opportunity to enjoy Sigmund Freud's personal direction.[1]

THE INITIAL PHASE

On October 16, Dorsey wrote to Freud himself, and just a few days later received confirmation that he was accepted for treatment. The analysis was to begin on October 23. Dorsey immediately informed Hans Maier, director of the Burghölzli Clinic in Zurich, that he was not staying and moved his family to Vienna within a matter of days. Dorsey had to take a taxi from the station to Freud's house to get there in time for his appointment. He was shown in by the maid and did not have to wait long.

> Professor Freud came out of an adjoining room, receiving me graciously with a friendly wave of his arm. Immediately I was aware of his alert presence. My reverent father transference began here. He bade me shed my topcoat and preceded me into another room where he was to interview me. . . . The Professor looked conservatively well dressed, a gold watch chain on his vest, wearing glasses. After brief amenities he said uncomplainingly that he had a bad cold and that he would prefer to begin my analysis on the following Monday. Opening conversation indicated to me that, had I not taken immediate advantage of his offered appointment, he would have withdrawn from the idea of working with me.[2]

In this first hour they agreed on the terms: the fee—100 schillings, or about $20 an hour—and the schedule—daily meetings except on Sundays and no vacation other than Christmas Day.[3] Dorsey was again very impressed by Freud's demeanor:

> [H]e seemed a very strong minded person of particular refinement. . . . His firm gait, station, posture or movement did not identify him specially with old age. His attention, interest, and general presence were that of a younger man than his short white beard and vanishing head of hair might suggest. . . . He spoke in a polite, quiet way, his English being clearly resourceful in depth and notably free of accent. . . . His lively gestures were easy and natural. I found pleasing, this neat, self-possessed, nice looking elderly gentlemen [sic] obviously wishing me to feel at ease and to get on with the business at hand. . . . He received a very prompt, workable, transference from me, impressing me in a fatherly manner as serious, kindly, and purposeful.[4]

After Dorsey had voiced his wishes about analysis and answered some questions concerning his career, Freud told him that he was going to analyze him. Dorsey was thrilled. At the end of the hour Freud said, "with very little seriousness"

> "By Monday I hope you will have learned German so that I can speak to you in German." . . . During my first *Stunde*, October 28 . . . I attempted free associating in my "broken" German and the Professor goodnaturedly found that "execrable," so with relief I proceeded in English.[5]

Freud cautioned Dorsey in this first interview not to take on anything extra during the initial phase of the treatment.

Dorsey was concerned about Freud's age and health from the start, the way he remembered being worried about his grandfather's physical well-being when he was little. In reality, the analysis was rarely interrupted, although Freud had to undergo at least two cancer operations in the course of their work together. Once Dorsey had a cold and suggested that it might be better to miss his appointment so that Freud would not catch it; but Freud, half irritated, replied that he did not need any special treatment. Dorsey also made allowances for possible memory lapses. When Freud learned this, he asked what evidence it was based on; Dorsey had to admit there was none. Furthermore, knowing Freud to be hard of hearing, Dorsey made a special effort to speak distinctly and loudly, and once jokingly commented that Freud was keeping him in analysis only because of his clear enunciation. Freud answered that he did not deny it. On the one hand, Dorsey wondered why Freud, whose time was precious and limited, had accepted him for treatment; on the other hand, he thought it befitting.

> My Professor Freud attained preeminently my revered father figure. I felt that the fact that I lived myself as his analysand was widely known and duly respected by each of my colleagues as well as by each one's chosen psychoanalyst. I quite naturally appreciated all of this privilege as being the just due of the youngest member of the most important family. It was like being born again.[6]

Dorsey began his first real hour by giving Freud an account of his childhood. Born in a small town in Iowa, he was the youngest of five. His father, who had grown up on a farm, made his living as a railroad supervisor. Dorsey described both parents as honest, simple, loving people and his childhood as peaceful and happy. He was named after the father of a family friend, John Morris, but decided to drop the second part of his name. When he mentioned his worry about this choice and the effect it might have had on his personality, Freud just replied that he was "not partial to 'Morris.' "[7] Religion, Dorsey recalled, had played an important part in his early upbringing but had not interfered with a strong sexual drive; he was always in love with one girl or another. He remembered in particular a very painful experience at age seven, when a girlfriend chose a new love after changing schools. During his adolescent years he was plagued by strong conflicts over masturbation, which he tried to resolve by suppressing his sexual impulses. In school Dorsey was successful both academically and socially, but he was bothered and humiliated by serious facial acne. The embarrassment over his face affected him greatly, and the topic came up at least once in a later analytic hour, when he wondered aloud what was the matter with him. Freud replied he might perhaps be thinking it was his face.

Dorsey had become interested in psychology in high school but remained undecided about a medical specialty until 1925, the beginning of his senior year in medical school. At that time—he was engaged to be married—he was offered a research position at the Iowa State Psychopathic Hospital under Dr. Orton, the director and a professor of psychiatry. During the next year, Dorsey researched certain processes and functions of the central nervous system and collaborated in the publication of studies in electrophysiology. When Orton left his post in 1927, Dorsey, at the age of 26, became the assistant director. The following year he accepted the post of assistant to Dr. Barrett, the director of psychiatry at the University of Michigan State Psychopathic Hospital. Because Barrett was more interested in the psychodynamic aspects of mental illness than Orton had been, a new dimension was added to Dorsey's primarily physiological orientation. After the publication of Dorsey's *Foundations of Human Nature* in 1935, he became Barrett's first associate professor.

Following the initial hour with Freud, Dorsey wrote in his journal that it had been "truly a soul-stirring experience. . . . Just to think of the father of psychoanalysis, being in the same room listening, correcting, always straightening and progressing."[8] He later realized that this description was more a reflection of his expectation of what was going to happen than an accurate portrayal of Freud's actual behavior.

> Certainly that was what I was expecting of my self analysis at the time. Fortunately it never happened. I profited immeasurably from the non-interfering and consciously self contained way in which the Professor conducted his work. . . . My psychoanalyst was not partial to comment, and commented so.[9]

Freud made it clear that the focus of their work was going to be on Dorsey's free associations. When in these early hours Dorsey asked a number of questions, Freud said:

> "Analysis based upon . . . free association must be a soliloquy—not a dialogue." [However, the Professor would often "answer" a question with that understanding reservation in it.] As he good humoredly put it: "Psychoanalysis is not a game of questions and answers, now, is it?"[10]

Notwithstanding this comment, Dorsey tried to get Freud to answer his questions—and sometimes succeeded. For example, he asked who Freud's favorite pupil was; Freud, without hesitation, said it was Karl Abraham. Another time Dorsey queried him on the importance of sexuality; Freud replied that sex is as important to a person's life as water is to chemistry.

Dorsey had little knowledge of psychoanalysis and wanted to learn about the theory from Freud. He was surprised about the process, in particular, the degree of Freud's inactivity. In the second week of the analysis, he asked Freud why he did not do or say more. This time Freud responded by telling a story about "the Japanese gardener who was reproached, after being hired, for sitting several days and doing no work; [he] rejoined that he *was* working, the first step in building the garden being to take in the landscape."[11]

Six weeks into the treatment Dorsey asked Freud what he thought about him. Freud replied that he found him very personal. When Dorsey criticized himself in the same hour for being slow with his associations to a dream, Freud reassured him, saying that it might take him a day longer.

Dorsey's portrayal of his analysis is more of a summary, anecdotal and focused on outside events, than a detailed and intimate account. He reveals little about the content of his hours with Freud; almost in passing and in very theoretical terms, he mentions that he and Freud discussed his oedipal wishes as well as screen memories of the primal scene. Dorsey notes in the preface that he originally kept the journal as a "professional log."[12] This may partially explain why the daily entries are concerned less with his treatment than with his thoughts on psychological theory, the lectures he attended at the University of Vienna and the Psychoanalytic Institute, and the people he was meeting. On the other hand, the journal may reflect a more general attitude or an attempt to screen out comments from Freud that punctured Dorsey's glorification of their relationship. Four months after they had begun working together, Freud commented on his patient's "pseudoscientific orientation and desire for further objective knowledge."[13] From a later vantage point, Dorsey wondered whether his preoccupation with the external environment was not a manifestation of resistance against the one thing Freud asked him to do—free-associate.

THE MIDDLE PHASE

Dorsey found free association difficult. He wrote later, at the end of January:

> My resistance was high but my consciousness for that fact was of an intellectual superficiality that defended it rather than enabled me otherwise to cope with it understandingly. Fortunately, the Professor understood that it was labor that only I could do. He obviously knew that his work was to see me insightfully through my difficult self-confrontation.[14]

Dorsey knew little about free association when he first came to Freud. Now he found out that it was going to be the main focus in his analysis. "Anew, full obedience about the importance of not withholding speaking of *any* mental content for any reason whatsoever, was my one psychoanalytic rule."[15] It took him a long time to learn. At first he avoided difficult topics or passed over quickly the meaning of what he was saying. But gradually he began to say everything that was on his mind—and to listen to it as well. Freud, who once likened Dorsey's associations to a "museum of psychopathology," let him know about his progress.[16] "The first time I practiced this kind of mind speaking from surface to depth (vertically as well as horizontally) the Professor observed, 'That is free association.' Happy day!"[17] One time, at the end of March, Freud rewarded him for having associated well by showing him a letter he thought would be of interest, in which an American psychoanalytic official asked Freud's help in deciding whether or not to admit a particular candidate to his psychoanalytic society.

Freud strictly monitored Dorsey's compliance to this rule. Although he found it difficult to speak his mind freely at first, Dorsey was later able to appreciate the advantage of the method and, in fact, measured the progress of his treatment by his ability to free-associate. Other than being encouraging to his patient when things were going well or consoling him that it might take a little more time, Freud had little help to offer.

> Once I spoke of the difficulty in free association. The Professor recalled complaining of an attack of dysentery he suffered during an American camping trip with Dr. James Putnam. The most help Dr. Putnam had to offer was, "That's too bad," observing that such an intestinal upset occurred often in foreigners. Professor Freud added genially that he had no more help to offer me than that.[18]

But it was not until later that Dorsey accepted the value of Freud's insistence on free association. At the time of his treatment he resisted it and continued to protest, directly or indirectly, about Freud's inactivity and his insistence that patients have to do the work of the analysis themselves.

The only thing Freud expected of Dorsey, besides speaking his mind freely, was that he respect the formal arrangements of the analysis. "Apart from doing my best to obey the psychoanalytic rule of speaking my mind without reservation so that I might observe it as such, I merely abided by the arrangements that made possible my free associations with the knowledge of his conscious presence."[19] These arrangements included arriving and leaving on time, lying on the couch, and paying the fee. Their work was rarely interrupted. Freud was extremely punctual; he never let Dorsey wait and never extended the treatment hour. Once, Dorsey requested a change of time. Freud agreed to it but told him that he had to work out the details with the patient whose hour he wanted.

On one occasion Dorsey was concerned about the privacy of his analytic hour. He had arisen from the couch to demonstrate a kind of gait and had noticed an open door. He was worried that someone might be overhearing his free associations. Dorsey once met Freud's wife, Martha: It had begun to rain during his therapy hour and she lent him a raincoat for the way back. He regularly saw Anna Freud at lectures and seminars organized through the Psychoanalytic Institute. And there was, as usual, a third party in the consulting room—Yofi. Freud told Dorsey that Yofi responded to the presence of resistance in a patient by leaving the room and that she indicated the end of the hour by getting up and yawning.

Once Freud remarked offhandedly that the only thing authors of current writings on mental health were proving was that they could read and write. Dorsey flinched upon hearing this, as he himself had published a book, which had received bad reviews. He wondered what Freud would think about it. When he mentioned his anguish over the bad reception of his book, Freud responded kindly, "Maybe it is not that bad."[20]

In general, Freud made what he said short and to the point and kept his interpretations decidedly tentative; Dorsey could take them or leave them.

> As to that much used term, interpretation, the Professor never tried to tell me anything about what I should or should not mean by any content in my free associating. Similarly, he certainly seemed free to speak his mind but only so that I might feel free to consider for myself what he might say.[21]

Dorsey characterized Freud's attitude as noninterfering. In response to questions he often remained vague and noncommittal. When Dorsey asked why he continued being so attached to women with long hair, Freud just said it was not time for the answer yet. In response to a question about why he did not repeat his statements for emphasis, Freud replied, "Like the lion, if my first pounce does not appear to work, I let it go at that."[22] Freud did not like the theoretical language of psychoanalysis. Rather, he kept his interpretations simple and once said that even the unconscious was "just a word."[23]

Despite the fact that Freud was less active and talkative than Dorsey might have wished, Dorsey did not think of him as uninvolved or withdrawn. On the contrary, he felt that Freud respected him and that he took every thought and association seriously: "The one word that characterized his analytic presence was: commitment. He practiced the finest tact in the form of ongoing attentiveness. . . . No loose work, no theorizing, no curing, no criticizing, no acting—just free interest."[24] He emphasized that Freud, while attentive, kind, and accepting, was not "supportive in the sense of countertransference; his strongest support was his dedication to the work."[25] Dorsey was also impressed with Freud's passion for truth. He was interested in all of Dorsey's free associations and had a habit of consulting books, dictionaries, and encyclopedias whenever a particular fact came into question. When there were disagreements between the two over some piece of knowledge, Freud always proved right; however, Dorsey never felt that Freud was showing him up.

At times, for all his seriousness and focus on the work, Freud could be funny and personable. He once leaned over the couch and sang Dorsey a few lines from Mozart's *Don Giovanni,* which was playing at the Vienna opera. Another time, when Dorsey had made some remark about Freud's father fixation, Freud said, "You may analyze me if you wish, but I shan't pay you for it."[26] For Christmas Freud gave his patient a copy of his recently published *New Introductory Lectures on Psycho-Analysis.*

Two months after the beginning of the analysis, Freud's physician, Max Schur, discovered a recurrence of Freud's cancer of the jaw and palate, which was surgically treated in January 1936. Despite Freud's serious health problems, Dorsey's treatment was only briefly interrupted. It was not until later that Dorsey realized how much Freud kept such difficulties to himself: "I am now exquisitely aware of what a tremendous effort his work must have been, but I knew absolutely nothing of the distress he must have been suffering at the time."[27] In February of 1936, Pichler found a leukoplakia that was removed in March.

From the beginning of the treatment, if not before, Freud had been Dorsey's hero. In early February, three months into the analysis, Dorsey was still very happy about being with him. "I am more than ever happy over my privileged opportunities for studying medical psychology [with him]. He is all that I hoped for."[28] There were, however, occasional hints of other feelings. In one of his first dreams, for instance, Dorsey found himself in the role of a "young and defenseless person being relentlessly pushed about by an inescapable man of great resourcefulness 'whom everybody knew' while large quantities of money seemed to be disappearing in the air."[29]

It is not clear from Dorsey's notes to what extent his reactions to Freud were analyzed. In discussing Freud's general reticence, Dorsey observes, "My analysis was a strictly personal, not inter-personal, experience."[30] This goes along with the following statement: "The Professor's method never encouraged me in the idea or feeling that anything was going on between us."[31] Dorsey uses the term *transference* primarily in reference to the oedipal relationship. A dream, actually a nightmare, in which he hangs on to a cliff with his hands while soldiers on horses ride over them, gave him a clue to understanding that aspect of his unconscious; when he presented this dream, which was traced back to his first disappointing love affair at age seven, Freud exclaimed, "What a classic Oedipus dream!"[32] Freud then interpreted Dorsey's relationship to the little girl as an attempt to sever the incestuous tie to his mother. This interpretation shed further light on his relationship to his father. "My ambivalent father transference resolved itself as I began to appreciate hate as hurt (inhibited) love."[33]

About three to four months into the analysis, Freud told Dorsey that it was time for him to start reading psychoanalytic literature. The analysand began with *The Question of Lay Analysis*. At the end of March Freud took him into his study and chose another book; he handed him *The Future of an Illusion* with the words, "This will start you on the road to Hades."[34] It appears that he made this choice in response to Dorsey's question about how psychoanalysis might affect his religious beliefs. Freud had replied that the book would help him understand the meaning of religion, a suggestion Dorsey later found useful.

Yet much as Dorsey admired Freud and felt privileged to be his patient, he was, by his own account, still struggling with tremendous resistance against free association. He wanted to focus his thoughts on theory, objective facts, and scientific knowledge and tried to engage Freud in a debate concerning the validity of psychoanalysis. Freud had little to say and even less help to offer. "When my resistance against free association surfaced as prejudice against psychoanalysis, Freud went along in a most helpfully resigned way, only once kindly saying, 'Oh, do I have to live through that again!' "[35]

In the middle of March, as Dorsey neared the completion of six months of treatment, he asked Freud how much longer the analysis would take. Up until this point, Dorsey had spoken only of his academic interest in psychoanalysis, as he was not planning to become an analyst himself. In response to the question, Freud told a story:

> "When the traveller came upon Aesop who was laboring on the road—breaking up stone—and asked him how long it was to the next town, say to Megara, Aesop responded, 'Go.' Angrily the traveller turned away and resumed his going. 'Three quarters of an hour,' called Aesop after him. The wayfarer asked, 'Why didn't you say so in the first place?' Aesop explained, 'I wanted to see just how you went, so that I could decide upon it.' "[36]

Dorsey later described this as yet another example of how Freud tried to teach him to find his own answers, but at the time it was given, this reply did not satisfy him. Several days later he again expressed his concern about how much longer he would have to be in analysis. This time Freud spoke "good naturedly of the American who boasted of making the complete tour of the Louvre in one hour and three quarters, and who then added, 'And if I'd had my rollerskates on I could have made it in an hour and a half.' "[37]

Dorsey realized only in hindsight how much he kept pressuring Freud to give him answers; Freud just as persistently refused to do so. It is not clear why the question of termination came up at this point and how it was decided that the analysis be continued. The money provided for his treatment by the Rockefeller grant was limited, but it appears that it paid for close to a year of treatment. With Freud's help, Dorsey was able to finance an additional month on his own, namely, by borrowing 2,500 schillings, equivalent to 25 hours of analysis, through Freud's son Martin, who was working in a bank.

THE TERMINATION PHASE

In the beginning of April, Dorsey received news from Michigan that Dr. Barrett, his supervisor, had suddenly died. This was unexpected and shocking on a personal level as well as in terms of its professional implications. Dorsey had hoped to replace Barrett one day as director of the University of Michigan State Psychopathic Hospital, and the training he was receiving during his sabbatical was geared toward that goal. Being only halfway through his time abroad and far away from the developments in Michigan, he began seeing his chances for this career advancement wane. The realization that he would have to change his plans affected his analysis deeply.

> No longer could I be satisfied to accept my analytic work as being only a theoretical addition to my pedagogical powers. Instead my compelling interest in its leading to my becoming a psychoanalyst started to take preference and pretty soon began to assume vital importance for me. All of this sharp turn of the direction of the goal of my analysis took the time that such growth requires. I was not aware of it at all for several weeks. . . . No doubt the Professor recognized this change in my expectation of what I wanted to derive from my analytic investment, but of course he was equal to it and dealt with it, like with all else, as part of the work. Regarding my troubled mind about Dr. Barrett's death he very kindly added, "It is the ones who are living who need the help."[38]

Until now Dorsey had been content and happy; Barrett's death made him depressed and anxious.

Although Dorsey wrote that this abrupt change in his career prospects and direction profoundly affected his analysis, it is not clear in precisely what way. He does comment in the journal that Freud's technique did not change as a result of it. In his notes he continues to dwell on the details of events outside the analysis—his classes at the institute, the people he met there, his thoughts on psychological theory, and the like. At the end of February he himself observed: "I notice the extent to which my journal notes deal with my living that I was accustomed to call (insightlessly) 'the external world,' not realizing that such self disregard was even happening! Even my positive transference was resistance!"[39] Dorsey later noted, also in retrospect, that he continued with this tendency even after he began to define his analysis as a personal rather than an academic endeavor. A comment from the journal at the beginning of May, in the seventh month of treatment, illustrates the way in which Dorsey's preoccupation with theory may have related to his personal concerns: "Psychoanalysis leads to the renunciations of infantilisms or, rather, to the proper expression of one's adulthood."[40] But he still was not ready to accept this insight on a deeper level and continued to hope that Freud would do the work for him. "Mark Twain resided in Vienna a while. I told the Professor a favorite story about him that I later understood to be a vehicle for my protest against waiting to be analyzed rather than facing my having to do it myself."[41] Most reluctantly, Dorsey finally began to accept more responsibility. At the end of July he wrote in his journal that he was beginning to resign himself to the fact that psychoanalysis was a "growing process."[42]

Freud turned 80 in May. Dorsey gave him some flowers and attended several events in his honor, all of which Freud avoided. At the end of the month the Freud family moved to Grinzing for the summer. Dorsey and his wife and children took up residence there also. It was a welcome change. He thought the quiet verdure of the little suburb was more appropriate for Freud and analysis than the city atmosphere had been. In the middle of July, Freud again missed a couple of days to have his jaw operated on. Dorsey wrote in his journal that the news made him sad. "When I learned later of the health hardships he had been undergoing, I marvelled at his ability to keep all of his difficulties integrated into the conduct of his work. The distinction is great: he had his health trouble, it did not have him."[43] Everyone returned to Vienna in the middle of September.

THE FINAL MONTH

In October, one month before the termination of his analysis, Dorsey visited several clinics in Germany to learn how mental health institutions were run on the continent. November 8 was his last day with Freud. After a little over a year of analysis, he was not prepared to leave.

> The time all too rapidly arrived that was set for termination of my free association with the Professor. . . . The actual stopping came hard. . . . I found the idea of being thrown back upon myself without my Professor,—a heavy burden involving painful self rejection including an intensive sense of failure. Since the death of my loyal and reliable friend, Dr. Barrett, I had been hoping desperately all along to attain my personal development as a fully disciplined psychoanalyst as soon as possible. I felt sure that Professor Freud could make me do it. The insurmountable truth remained: I seemed unable to do it, without growing further helpfulness for that doing.[44]

In his journal Dorsey emphasizes his worry about the training part of his analysis coming to an end and leaving him ill equipped to do analytic work.

> My psychoanalytic status seemed unbearable, that of its being finished but myself not yet ready to belong to it officially in the sense of continuing training essential for my qualifying as a practicing psycho-analyst. . . . I began to realize that I must renounce my unspoken but powerful phantasy of having my Professor Freud omnipotently make a psychoanalyst out of me. He had done all he could.[45]

Only in passing does Dorsey mention his sadness over the fact that a year of feeling secure had come to an end.

Toward the end of his treatment with Freud, Dorsey asked what, in his opinion, had helped the most to elucidate the nature of his dynamics. Without hesitation, Freud reminded him of the dream that had revealed the vicissitudes of his oedipal conflicts. He had always made it clear that he thought of the work with dreams as the most relevant.

Dorsey still had about six months of his sabbatical left. He decided to continue in analysis with someone less expensive than Freud, prefer-ably a woman. He discussed this with Freud, who listened and then suggested Heinz Hartmann. Dorsey took his advice; he liked the idea of working with Hartmann, whom he considered a sort of younger brother to Freud. In this way, too, perhaps, Dorsey could remain in the family and in the privileged position of littlest. After several more months in analysis with Hartmann, Dorsey prepared to return to the United States. The work with Freud, he wrote later, remained one of the highlights of his life; as a person and clinician, Freud had affected him profoundly.

Freud's Analysis
of Smiley Blanton

SMILEY Blanton was born on May 7, 1882, in Unionville, Tennessee, the son of Hiram and Sally (née Brunson). He did his undergraduate work at Vanderbilt University in Nashville and received his M.D. degree from Cornell University in Ithaca, New York. At 28, Blanton married Margaret Gray. Between 1916 and 1928 he held hospital and medical school psychiatry positions at Johns Hopkins, the University of Wisconsin, the University of Minnesota, and Vassar College. During World War I, he completed a tour of duty with the Army Medical Corps both in the United States and overseas. Despite these early accomplishments, it was not until his late 40s, following an analysis with Freud, that Blanton found a calling, one to which he devoted the remainder of his life—the integration of psychiatry and religion.

In 1937, Blanton and the Reverend Norman Vincent Peale opened the Religio-Psychiatric Clinic of the Marble Collegiate Church in New York City to offer free Christian psychiatry to people suffering from emotional problems. In 1951, Blanton and Peale formed the American Foundation of Religion and Psychiatry so that a training program in pastoral counseling could be added to the clinic. In addition to coauthoring earlier works in speech pathology with his wife, Blanton collaborated with Peale in the writing of two books—*Faith Is the Answer: A Pastor and a Psychiatrist Discuss Your Problems* and *The Art of Real Happiness*. At 73, he put forth his view, in *Love or Perish*, that mental illness results from the failure to approach life in a loving, constructive way. He died on October 30, 1966. Blanton was 47 when the analysis began; Freud was 73. All of the following quotes are from Blanton's book *Diary of My Analysis with Sigmund Freud*, unless otherwise indicated.

In his relations with Freud, Blanton was at pains to be friendly, appreciative, and unprickly. These soon appear to be reaction formations—presumably, ones that were later pressed into service in his theories about the necessity of Christian love. Blanton was desperate to avoid appearing resistant and was terrified that resistance would be unmistakably revealed by his being late for appointments. Apparently, he imagined himself the victim of robbery by Freud and thus was overly scrupulous about their financial arrangements and paid early. Underneath his eager, if adulterated, compliance, Blanton seems combative, even nationalistically chauvinistic—as if he felt himself to be the Protestant Yankee pitted against a German-Jewish Freud. He supplies dream after dream in an apparent attempt to keep himself (his conscious being) divorced from unsavory and dangerous proceedings.

What is most striking is how unwelcome and warded off this middle-aged psychiatrist's resistance and rivalry were and how desperately he clung to what appears to have been a religious grandmaternal transference in defense against a negative paternal one. Despite Freud's advanced age, Blanton returned to him again and again, like a Christian pilgrim in search of a miracle cure, until one wonders if even Freud's death would have been sufficient to deter Blanton from further requests for analytic renewal.

Blanton appears genuinely to have been a decent fellow who was merely trying to be better than a person can be; after all, good manners—when they are not false gestures and empty formalities—do show respect and can be pleasing. Thus, Freud responded to Blanton's strained efforts to cooperate in a gentle and patient manner. He gave Blanton books to read, urged him to associate freely, reassured him that he was not responsible for the nasty contents of his unconscious mind, helped him with his career, and tried to interpret the transference, both in its past and current aspects. Perhaps in the final few years of his life Freud was resigning himself to the fate of a European cultural treasure destined to be plundered by souvenir hunters and appreciated the fact that this one at least was trying to be friendly about it.

*   *   *

THE INITIAL PHASE

Smiley Blanton was 20 minutes late for his first appointment with Freud on September 1, 1929. He had taken a taxi from his hotel in Berchtesgaden to the villa just outside of town where Freud was spending the summer with his family. The thought of beginning his analysis by making Freud wait was mortifying, but at least he was not to blame. The driver knew the area less well than he had claimed and got lost. Finally they arrived. Blanton knocked timidly on the front door that stood ajar.

> After a wait of two or three minutes, I heard someone moving in the room just off the hall. A few seconds later, a frail, small-statured, gray-haired man with a gray beard appeared in the hallway and came toward me. Although he looked older than in the photographs I had seen, I recognized the approaching figure to be that of Freud himself. He was carrying a cigar in his hand, and there was something almost diffident in his manner as he addressed me. "Is this Doctor Blanton?" he said in a low voice. His articulation was somewhat indistinct, doubtless due to the operations he has undergone for cancer of the upper right jawbone. When I replied in the affirmative, he added, "I thought the appointment was at three o'clock."[1]

Freud did not seem irritated as much as surprised to be kept waiting by his new patient. On the way to the consulting room, Blanton hastened to explain the reason for his delay and then handed Freud a letter of introduction from the American patient whose hour he was taking. Freud, after reading the letter, indicated that he should lie on the couch and then asked him what he knew about how psychoanalysis was prac-ticed. Half-sitting on the couch, Blanton mentioned, among other things, that the patient should be relaxed and speak his mind as freely as possible.

> "Well, then," said Freud, "why don't you relax?" I stretched out in a more comfortable position. . . . After I had relaxed, Freud said, "You may wonder why I make so few comments, or help you so little." I then began to give Freud the thoughts that were in my mind.[2]

Blanton told Freud that he regretted being late, that he was glad to be in analysis with him, and that he had always preferred him over Adler and Jung. Freud asked why, but Blanton could not explain the reasons. He went on to speak of feeling insecure about his life and began to describe his background.[3]

Blanton was born and grew up in Tennessee. His mother died of tuberculosis when he was still young; shortly thereafter, his father married her sister. As an only child, Blanton was the center of attention in the household, which consisted of his parents, uncle, grandparents, and two black servants. He idealized his grandmother, an aggressive and control-ling woman who was very critical of him and pushed him to live up to her standards. With his father he had little in common. In his own estimation he was badly spoiled, but others saw him as "overcontrolled, overmanaged, overloved."[4] Being extremely tenacious and stubborn, Blanton had few friends. In school he did not get along with his peers or teachers and was only a marginal student; his main interests were English and history.

Contrary to everyone's expectations, however, Blanton was accepted to Vanderbilt University, from which he barely graduated with a bachelor of science degree. Even though his academic performance was mediocre, he was accepted into the graduate program in English at Harvard. He also enrolled in a drama school, where he became interested in stuttering and speech defects. From there, his interests evolved to medicine and psychiatry. At age 27, Blanton met his wife, and they married one year later. He graduated from Cornell University Medical School at 32. From 1914 to 1924 the couple lived in Wisconsin, where Blanton had established a speech and mental hygiene clinic in the Department of Public Speaking at the state university. During this time he went to various psychiatric hospitals for further training and served in World War I as a psychiatrist. In 1924, he went to Minneapolis, where he started a child guidance clinic in the public schools. He left there in 1927 to organize and direct a nursery school that was being opened at Vassar and to teach courses at the college. He was now on a 12-month leave of absence from Vassar to study psychoanalysis in Vienna.

Blanton was impressed with Freud's presence after the first hour:

> At all times he seemed in close touch with what I was saying. I felt he was interested, that he was taking in what I was giving him. There was none of that cold detachment which I had imagined was the attitude an analyst is supposed to take. As we went along, Freud's simple manner made me feel secure and easy. At the same time, there was a detachment which was not repelling but pleasant.[5]

He also wrote:

> The impressions that stand out after this first meeting are Freud's smallness of stature (about 5′ 4″, I should judge), his soft and almost deprecating manner, the way in which he makes you feel at ease yet combines this with a detachment which leaves you free to express yourself.[6]

Freud was 5′ 7″.

When Blanton heard a clock strike four, he stopped in the middle of his sentence and got up. Freud said he regretted that the hour had been so short. Blanton asked when Freud was planning to return to Vienna.

He was going to leave in the middle of September, Freud replied, but would first go to Berlin for a month; if he wanted to, Blanton could come with him. Blanton agreed to accompany him there and then left.

Blanton made sure not to be late again; he arrived for his next session half an hour early and waited outside until Freud summoned him. This time he went straight to the couch and lay down. Freud encouraged him to treat this hour like a new one, not as a sequel to the preceding one. Before his appointment Blanton had developed colitis and in addition had cut his finger. He now wondered whether these physical symptoms were a sign of resistance. There was more than one way of understanding this kind of symptom, Freud replied, and resistance was only one of them. Blanton returned to the question from the day before of why he preferred Freud over Adler and Jung. He explained that he admired in Freud the combination of artist and scientist, that he did not like the moral underpinnings in Jung's theories, and that he thought Adler received credit for ideas that were not originally his. Which of his writings had he read? Freud asked, and which of Jung's and Adler's? Blanton answered that he had read all of Freud's works that had been translated into English; he then continued with his account of his childhood and training. Freud interrupted: "Have you prepared this?"

> Yes, I replied. "But," said Freud, "you must not prepare what you are to say but give freely what comes into your mind. That is the classical method." I was silent for several moments—whereupon Freud said, "You may go ahead and give me what you have prepared!"[7]

Freud wanted to know whether Blanton had any children and when he heard that he did not, he expressed his sympathy. He did have a dog, Blanton said, to whom he was very attached. Freud agreed that the feelings for dogs and children are similar, except for the lack of ambivalence in the relationship to animals. Blanton argued that one could feel hostile toward animals as well but did not pursue the point when Freud insisted on his idea. Blanton spoke more about his personality and preferences, and the hour was up. In the wake of this second appointment, he felt somewhat depressed and disappointed without knowing quite why. It was perhaps, he thought, the prospect of soon confronting his problems. Also, he felt bad about having trouble understanding Freud, whose speech after several operations on his mouth and jaw was less than clear. Blanton tried to console himself with the thought that his difficulty was a product of resistance that, he hoped, would lessen after a while.

The fear of being late still haunted Blanton. He notes in his journal that he had to run to make it on time for his third appointment. Freud asked him whether he had prepared any topics. Even though it was hard,

Blanton replied, he had managed to resist the temptation. He went on to talk about his prejudice against Germans, which he deplored, as he did the general level of hatred in the world. Since he was speaking very fast and in English, Freud could not follow what he was saying and told him he needed to slow down. Blanton next talked about his wife, Margaret, and their unhappiness about not having children. Freud was interested to hear more about his wife and asked several questions about her. Among other things, Blanton explained, she was doing research on the female orgasm; she had also just started her psychoanalysis with Clara Thompson. Freud was pleased when he heard that Thompson had been analyzed by Ferenczi. At the end of the hour Freud commented that he was associating better: "Freud rose and said, 'It was much better. You were much freer than before,' and bowed me out."[8]

Blanton arrived for his next hour hungry, tired, and in discomfort from colitis. It surprised him that Freud did not interpret his physical symptoms as resistance. On the contrary, he suggested that it might be caused by the heat. Blanton's bad mood dissolved with Freud's kindness and interest. As he wrote in his journal: "Freud was especially gracious. I think he likes me and finds me interesting. In fact, he said so—'It is very interesting'—when I was through today."[9] When Blanton talked about his financial situation, saying that he had saved up $20,000, Freud remarked that this was his anal side and added that when he was his age, he did not have as much. Blanton admitted that he was a little worried to let Freud know about his savings for fear he might be charged a higher fee than the current $25 an hour, but Freud only reminded him to not allow his fears to interfere with his associations.

Next Blanton talked in greater detail about his career plans. He was not satisfied with his work at Vassar College; he found the program too restrictive. It was now his wish to become a psychoanalyst. Freud observed, "I have been astonished at your frequent changes [of residence]. I should have thought that with your feeling of insecurity you would have remained in one place."[10] Blanton went on to express his misgivings about incompetent doctors who were earning money; he mentioned one by name. Freud knew the person in question and gave an interpretation of how the doctor's manic–depressive illness affected the running of his private practice. In the course of this hour Blanton told Freud how grateful he was about being able to work with him. Freud replied that Dr. Amsden—a friend of Blanton's from Johns Hopkins and Vassar who went into analysis with Ferenczi—had recommended him so highly that he was glad to accept him. As for himself, Blanton continued, he had sacrificed a lot for this analysis. Freud said he was aware of it and hoped it would be worth his while. Shortly before four o'clock, with five minutes left, Blanton got up. "As you will," said Freud, spreading out his hands, and then adding, "That is very interesting. You must be patient. We will get to the deeper layers, and then I shall not be so silent, I shall give more of myself."[11]

In the following hour, toward the end of the first week of the analysis, Freud seemed bored. When Blanton began to criticize himself for being infantile, Freud interpreted these self-reproaches as a sign of resistance. His observation was confirmed by more evidence later on.

> [Freud asked,] "May I ask you an indiscreet question: How do you sleep at night?" I replied that I slept poorly, waking up every two hours throughout the night. "Do you dream?" "Yes, frequently. I had a dream last night." "Why did you not tell it?" "Because I wanted to wait until I could write it down as soon as I awakened," I replied. "But you must not do this," said Freud. "To write the dream down increases the resistance, so that it is often impossible to analyze it. No. Do not write the dream down. If the resistance takes it away, let it do so."[12]

Blanton wanted to discuss a dream he had had a while ago, but Freud interrupted him and said that only more recent ones would be useful. As Blanton was leaving, Freud said, "For an analyst not to tell his dreams is a nice bit of resistance!"[13] In the course of the hour Blanton had expressed his sympathy for poor people and had then wondered whether it was a compensation for his sadism, but he had concluded, and Freud agreed, that at least in part it must be genuine.

Since there had not been enough time the previous hour, Blanton discussed his most recent dream the next day. To Freud's question about why he thought he had so much resistance, Blanton responded that he did not know and wondered aloud if it perhaps had to do with sexuality. But Freud had something else in mind; he suggested that the resistance had to do with the treatment, a connection that occurred to him because Blanton had dreamed about a car, a frequent symbol of psychoanalysis. Blanton reluctantly agreed. It was difficult to imagine, he said, that he would perceive Freud so negatively. But then, after giving it more thought, he wondered whether perhaps he was worried about not getting from Freud what he was hoping for. This time Freud agreed. Blanton felt comfortable with him, "Again I am impressed by Freud's soft and easy manner. He does not push you. He does not make emphatic statements often. When he does, it is in a very undominating manner."[14]

In the following hour Blanton recalled certain unpleasant things he had done in the past, which he then tried to justify. Freud interrupted and told him not to try to explain the reasons; they would become clear soon enough. He quoted Oliver Cromwell: "You never get so high as when you don't know where you are going." This maxim, Freud said, was applicable to psychoanalysis as well. Still, Blanton felt that his actions deserved being defended by the circumstances; otherwise, they might create the wrong impression. But Freud insisted, "It is the fact that is important, is it not?"[15]

Both analyst and patient agreed that the flow of associations continued to be hampered by strong resistance. Freud gave advice on how to deal with it. "The way to treat resistance . . . is to let it grow until it defeats itself. Today has been absolutely sterile. . . . It takes time to develop the right attitude and to overcome resistance. But I am sure you will be of much assistance in helping us to overcome it."[16] It had surprised Blanton from the beginning that Freud did not offer much help and that he sometimes did not speak at all for 10 or 15 minutes. He found it difficult to get used to. In the meantime, he kept bringing in dreams, one of which expressed his fear of psychoanalysis. He showed Freud an American newspaper clipping about Adler, which sparked a discussion about the psychoanalytic movement, its renegades, and its future.

As they went along, Freud taught Blanton the essentials of psychoanalytic technique. Two weeks into the treatment, for instance, Freud talked much of the hour about resistance and free association. He said that the analyst should never try to understand exactly what the patient means but should be satisfied with helping the patient overcome his resistance so he could figure things out for himself; forcing the matter would only heighten the *Widerstand*. When Blanton was reluctant to give his associations to a dream, Freud continued his lecture:

> "May I give you what seems to be a rule of analysis?" He then repeated the admonition about giving free reign to the unconscious, without reservations. "You are not responsible for your unconscious," he said. "But while you are bringing up the material, you must not have any moral judgments about it. . . . [I]t is only when you have laid self-criticism aside, and when you do not care what the analyst thinks, that you are able to get at the depth of the unconscious. Self-criticism is a form of inhibition. And excuses for the unconscious may lead to insecurity. For it is only a step from excusing the material from the unconscious to being insecure in telling what is in the unconscious."[17]

In the middle of September, two weeks after they had begun working together, Freud went to Berlin to have his dental plate repaired. Blanton followed him along with his wife, who had the opportunity there of meeting Freud herself. Even though the visit lasted only five minutes, Margaret was greatly impressed with Freud and with what she perceived to be his capacity to get at the truth. The sojourn in Berlin lasted longer than originally planned; they all returned to Vienna at the end of October. No journal entries are available from this time period.

THE MIDDLE PHASE

Blanton continued to bring new dreams to his analysis. Finally, after about eight weeks, Freud had had enough: "Are you not fed up with dreams? You need to give also what is in your conscious mind."[18] Blanton complained that psychoanalysis was a difficult enterprise. That difficulty, Freud retorted, was common in people who either were analysts themselves or knew the literature. He explained as follows:

> "They lack naïveté. The analyst should realize that the unconscious mind does not have the opposites that the conscious mind has. . . . It is necessary for the unconscious to express itself freely. When we find unmoral attitudes or qualities, do not try to bring out their opposites. Let us appreciate that we are unmoral, savage beings in the unconscious."[19]

Eventually, he continued, the contradictions between values in the conscious and impulses in the unconscious would resolve themselves, but this should not be attempted too soon so as not to hamper the expression of the unconscious. For some reason there are no journal entries from November 9, 1929, until January 22, 1930.

Three months into the treatment, the subject of Shakespeare's plays came up. Freud very much startled Blanton when he asked him whether he believed Shakespeare to be the man who had written the plays. Blanton, who considered himself somewhat of an expert—he had been an English and drama major for 12 years, had acted in some of Shakespeare's plays, and had memorized a number of them—answered in the affirmative. When Freud gave him a book whose author claimed that it was not Shakespeare who had written the plays, Blanton was shaken up. "I was very much upset. I thought to myself that if Freud believes Bacon or Ben Jonson or anyone else wrote Shakespeare's plays, I would not have any confidence in his judgment and could not go on with my analysis. So I asked my wife to read the book and tell me what she thought."[20] It was only after Margaret had read the book and found it to be a serious and scholarly work that Blanton himself studied it. He agreed with her, even though he was not swayed by the writer's reasoning. His obviously shaky faith in Freud was reinstated, and the crisis was over.

The journal notes resume at the end of January. Blanton was reading *The Interpretation of Dreams,* and he told Freud how dramatic he found the circumstances under which it was written—the poor Jewish doctor who was willing to risk everything for his beliefs. In his opinion, Blanton ventured to say, opening the book with "I shall prove . . . " was comparable to the greatest works ever, such as those of Descartes and St. Paul. Freud responded that it had not seemed heroic to him then, but he agreed with Blanton that the theses he had put forth in the book had remained essentially unaltered even in the current eighth edition.

Blanton then spoke about a class on mental hygiene he was going to teach at Vassar in the summer and was wondering how not to be superficial when lecturing on the subject of psychoanalysis. Freud cautioned against remaining too much on the surface. He used Adler's theory of the inferiority complex to demonstrate the uselessness of a theory that misses the most essential point, namely, that the child feels inferior not because it has inferior organs but because it is unloved. The difficulty for parents in raising children, Freud continued, lies in finding the right balance between being loving and frustrating. Freud also noted the danger of parents projecting their own wishes and fantasies onto the child. Apropos of a remark by Blanton that teachers frequently hate their children, Freud said that hate must be replaced by love, except that there are certain instances, such as penis envy and castration anxiety, where hate plays an important role and must be identified correctly. On the subject of women, Freud said that all girls identify with their mothers yet in cases where the relationship is hostile the identification may not announce itself until later in life. Freud added that when the bride is a virgin, there often occurs a change in her personality after she marries. For these reasons, Freud said, it is hard for men to predict women's personalities in the future: "Picking a wife is one of the most difficult things in this civilization."[21]

Five and a half months into the analysis, Freud gave Blanton a set of his *Collected Papers* as a gift. This was prompted by a remark by Blanton that he was saving up money to buy Freud's books. Following this, the patient dreamed about war, soldiers defending a railway station, and a dog pulling a box filled with cartridges through rows of pillars that were supporting the roof. His associations revealed the connection to Freud's gift: He remembered that during the war he had fought against the Germans over a railroad station; he linked that battle to the struggle between psychoanalysis and its dissidents. Another memory established the association between Freud's gift and the boxes of cartridges in the dream: He recalled building boxes to have his books moved; the pillars holding up the roof made him think of society and the kind of collapse Freud's theories would cause if their true meaning were understood. In another dream Blanton found himself quoting Shakespeare; these associations, too, returned to Freud's books. When over a period of several days his patient's dreams became increasingly difficult to interpret, Freud said, "For the past few days . . . your dreams have been growing more and more obscure. This can have only one meaning: There is a change in the transference. It is probably due to the present of the books. You will see from this what difficulties gifts in analysis always make."[22]

When Freud was not giving books to Blanton, he was loaning them to him. One was a book by Roback on the contribution of Jews to art, literature, and the sciences. Even though he did not think it was very good—he detested the kind of inaccuracies in the section on psychoanalysis—he knew that Blanton would be interested in the subject. Blanton, after reading it, agreed with Freud's opinion of the book and asked him what he thought about the theory that psychoanalysis was a Jewish science. Freud said that being Jewish had helped him only insofar as it was a preparation for being an outcast but that otherwise psychoanalysis was a science and not the product of a particular cultural or religious belief system. He admitted that it had worried him at one time that people would make this connection; for that reason he had tried to make Jung president of the International Association of Psychoanalysis. In another paper Freud gave Blanton to read, the same author, Roback, criticized his theory of slips of the tongue.

It was the end of February and of six months of analysis. Blanton arrived again several minutes late for his appointment. He had cut the time a little close and was unable to get a taxi right away. His tardiness upset him a great deal.

> I was quite flustered about it. When I went into the waiting-room, the outside door to the consulting room was open, but the inside door was closed. The maid asked me to go in. Freud was in his library, smoking. He was quite composed and kindly, as though I had not been late, but I was still flustered. As I lay down, I pulled out my watch and said, "I am afraid my watch is a little slow. I had best set it by yours." "My watch is usually right," he replied, but he did not give me the time. Instead he asked, "You were at dancing school?" "Yes," I said. "I left at ten minutes of six but could not get a taxi at once." Freud said no more, and I began my analysis.[23]

Later in the hour Freud referred to the paper by Roback, saying that Blanton perhaps agreed with some of the criticisms leveled against his theories. As for himself, he added, he thought the paper was silly; it contained several inaccurate statements about him and about psychoanalysis, inaccuracies that discredited the paper as a serious piece of writing in his eyes.

Several days later, toward the end of an hour, Blanton spoke about a dream. Freud was particularly interested in it and asked him to continue with his associations the following day. In the dream a Methodist preacher shows Blanton a church he has built that is "compact but stupidly designed."[24] It has only one door, and its two steps function simultaneously as stools for adults and children. Inside, rich decorations cover the walls and a veil is draped over the ceiling. On the veil are painted clouds, through which shine rays of light. There is a tank; it has a small bathtub or coffin for immersion but is broken and too small to be used. Through his associations Blanton understood the dream to be an expression of a criticism toward psychoanalysis, symbolized by the poorly constructed church. In particular, he disliked its emphasis on anality and the fact that only very intelligent people could make use of it. He added that the decorations were put in to make it less barren. Freud had some further ideas.

> "You see," Freud commented, "you can never tell what a thing means until you have associated to it." (This is too strong; he said "often," not "never.") "In one case, decorations might mean something else. The veil and the lights mean that analysis has taken away heaven. And the broken tank means circumcision. It is really a Jew that has built the house and is showing you about."[25]

Blanton went on to say that in his opinion it was simplistic to reduce a person's choice of career to a matter of compensation. Freud agreed that there could be other reasons for making a particular career choice; he maintained that in the case of a surgeon, for example, sublimation was an intrinsic component. For psychiatrists, Freud added, the psychological motivation was a fear of not being normal. At times, however, a career choice is, he allowed, more a product of circumstance than of active pursuit; Wagner-Jauregg, for instance, became a psychiatrist, and an excellent one at that, only because he was not accepted in any other hospital department. "He does not fulfill my theory," Freud concluded.[26]

THE TERMINATION PHASE

As noted, it was Freud's custom to have his patients pay their bill at the end of the month. In March, Blanton still owed $150 for February. Freud preferred to be paid in dollars by his American patients, because it was a more stable currency than the Austrian schilling. Getting the foreign money, however, was often difficult and sometimes caused a delay in paying. When Blanton finally received his money in the first week of March, he not only brought Freud the $150 he owed but also gave him

$350 in advance. Freud had qualms about accepting money for services not yet rendered.

> As he took it, he said, "You must promise to ask for a return of this from my family in case of my premature death." Once before, when I paid him $100 in advance, he had said the same thing. I asked him at that time if he had any reason to think that he might die suddenly. "No special reason," he had replied. . . . "I think about the possibility of death every day. It is good practice."[27]

At the end of the hour, Freud suggested that Blanton might have more to say about his thoughts on psychoanalysis. This comment prompted two dreams the following night. In the first dream Blanton is talking to Freud face-to-face. They are interrupted twice by people coming into the room. Blanton feels that he is being cheated out of his money by a badly conducted psychoanalysis. In the second dream Blanton is to speak to a group of people about psychoanalysis and education. The realization that Freud, who is present in another room, can hear makes him very self-conscious. Blanton believed the first dream expressed his criticism toward analyses that strayed from the rules. He had been having conversations with colleagues about the importance of such technical devices as the couch, conversations in which he defended the psychoanalytic position set forth by Freud. Just the day before, Freud had talked about his papers on technique:

> "I feel that they are entirely inadequate. I do not believe that one can give the methods of technique through papers. It must be done by personal teaching. Of course, beginners probably need something to start with. . . . But if they follow the directions conscientiously, they will soon find themselves in trouble. Then they must learn to develop their own technique."[28]

Blanton thought the second dream concerned his doubt as to whether he was able to give a favorable presentation of psychoanalysis. Freud told him that Blanton's hopes of having psychoanalysis accepted might be too high. He had to realize it was the subject itself, like the very existence of the unconscious, that created resistance. And if a choice had to be made between making psychoanalysis palatable to Americans by diluting its ideas (as Jung had suggested) or having it rejected, Freud continued, he would choose to stay with the unmitigated truth.

It was almost the end of March now. In one of their many discussions of psychoanalytic theory, Blanton talked about Freud's paper "A Child Is Being Beaten," from which he gathered that the child first acquires a feeling of sin from the Oedipus complex and then transfers it to masturbation. Freud argued that a feeling of sin could be obtained in other ways and asked when the paper was written; it turned out that Blanton had misread the date by nine years. Freud suggested that in the future he should be more careful when reading psychoanalytic literature. "It is just this which the critics fail to do. They seem to think that analysis was dropped from heaven or erupted from hell—that it is fixed like a block of lava and not a body of facts which have [sic] been slowly and painfully gathered by scientific research."[29] Freud pointed out that psychoanalytic theory was constantly being revised. For instance, he said, the Oedipus complex was still considered central in the neuroses of men, but in the case of women there was now an indication that the source of the neurosis, namely, her attachment to the mother, occurred at an earlier point in development.[30] He acknowledged that the development of the girl was much more complicated than that of the boy.

In a later hour Freud talked about some gender differences: It was a particular characteristic of women to become unavailable to psycho-analysis once they got involved in a love affair whereas male analysands could continue pursuing other activities. With boys he noticed a strong tendency to turn active into passive. Freud also told Blanton about new physiological research concerning children's sexuality that confirmed psychoanalytic findings, namely, that the sex organs of children at birth are well developed and that this development continues for a couple of years, after which point a regression occurs. He was interested to hear that Blanton's wife had found that newborn boys have erections.

When necessary, Freud reminded Blanton to free-associate: "You must follow the rule of analysis and be free to let your mind go as it will. Do not feel that you must keep along some preconceived path. You will probably get where you are going just the same. The analyst must follow where you go."[31] Later in the hour he gave an example of what can happen when the analyst does not follow the patient's lead: Early in his career he told a woman patient in the very first session that he did not believe she was as happily married as she had told him. She returned the following day and said that she realized he was right and that she therefore did not require any more treatment. With that, she left the hour—and psycho-analysis.

In the middle of April, Freud suggested that Blanton try to sleep on his back or side rather than on his stomach, a habit he thought probably had its origin in childhood. The analysis of Blanton's dreams was an important part of their work, and it appears that Freud advised this change in position as part of that effort.[32] Several days later the following incident involving Freud's dog gave rise to a dream: "The last two nights Freud has had his chow dog in the room. Two nights ago, as he came out of his hour with Dr. Jackson, he ran through the hall like a boy, expecting the dog to follow. But Dr. Jackson (she was just leaving) spoke to the dog, and the dog remained to speak to her."[33] In the dream Blanton's own dog, Bobs, finds a porcupine in a hollow tree. He throws it out of its hiding place and then swallows it. Blanton cuts it out from the dog's throat and in the process some quills get stuck in his thumb. The dream made him think about the story a doctor friend had just told him: A mother brought in her baby, who had been crying for a long time; it was finally discovered that the child's thumb was swollen. This led to another association about babies: the myth that they come from hollow stumps. Two quotes from Shakespeare occurred to Blanton in this context: the "fretful porcupine" from *Hamlet* and "untimely ripped from his mother's womb," a phrase he thought was from *Julius Caesar*.[34] Bothered as always by inaccuracies and factual misinformation, Freud corrected him with regard to the latter quote, saying that the statement was made in reference to Macduff and was from *Macbeth*. Blanton was once again astounded at the scope of Freud's knowledge. But Freud also had an association of his own to Blanton's dream:

> Mention of the porcupine led Freud to say, "When I was asked to go to America in 1909, I did not expect much, but I wanted to see a porcupine. In the Adirondacks, I saw a dead one. When I got back, Dr. Ferenczi gave me this little model." Whereupon he went into his room and brought out a small model of a porcupine for me to see. We spoke of its habits, then went on with the associations to my dream.[35]

Toward the end of April there was a short break in the analysis. Blanton went to Budapest for a few days to meet with Ferenczi to discuss with him his interest in stuttering. The problem fascinated him, and he often brought it up during his therapy hours. But Freud did not have much to say about it. His only thought was that it appeared to be a combination of oral eroticism and constitution. In the first hour after his return to Vienna on April 23, Blanton reported that he had read some critical reviews of Freud's new work, *Civilization and Its Discontents*. Freud repudiated these criticisms, saying that the authors could not have read the book since the English translation had not yet appeared. Blanton then spoke of a particular patient of Ferenczi's who had developed a negative transference; he added that, by contrast, his own transference to Freud was not negative. But Freud was not entirely convinced.

> "There is just one thing—perhaps I should not mention it," Freud remarked, "but I will give it to you for what it is worth. Perhaps you have not been entirely frank. It sometimes happens that a patient makes a mental reservation, which is easy to do, and then the analysis

goes on happily and smoothly, with little or no negative transference."[36]

Blanton asked whether he was referring to anything in particular that might indicate the presence of a negative transference, but Freud replied that he had mentioned it merely as a possibility—although, he added, Blanton's general tendency to be very positive might raise a certain doubt. What would happen in the case of a person who is reasonably justified in holding back some information, such as a priest? Blanton inquired. Freud answered that he once treated a diplomat who complained of problems in the presence of authorities. This patient insisted that, owing to the secretive nature of his position, he could not divulge any details about his work. Freud treated him with some success but felt that the results would have been better if the patient had not been allowed to hide behind his secrets.

It appears that this was the last regular meeting for a while. On April 24, Freud was hospitalized in Vienna for treatment of a heart condition. After his discharge on May 4, he returned to the Berlin sanatorium for further work on his mouth prosthesis. Blanton followed Freud to Germany, as he had done the year before, and met with him, albeit irregularly, until June. There are no journal entries from the time in Berlin except for the last session, and in the previous notes no reference is made to Freud's upcoming hospitalizations.

Blanton was due back at Vassar to teach summer school. His last meeting with Freud, on June 30 in the Berlin sanatorium, lasted only a few minutes. Freud gave him a letter of introduction to Ernest Jones, whom Blanton was planning to visit in London before returning to the United States. In their meeting on April 24, before Freud's leave from their regular analytic work, Blanton had mentioned the idea of continuing his analytic work with A. A. Brill in New York. This intention had met with Freud's full approval, and Blanton now told him that he had decided on Brill. He then asked Freud whether he thought he would be ready after one more year with Brill to begin practicing psychoanalysis. In Freud's opinion, that estimate was reasonable. He added, "I don't think you are neurotic."[37]

A FIRST RESUMPTION

Five years later Blanton returned to Vienna and to Freud for two more weeks of analysis; he was now 53, Freud 79. On August 3, 1935, shortly after his arrival, Anna gave him an appointment with her father for the same day at four o'clock. This year the Freud family was again spending the summer in Grinzing. Blanton was still frantic about being punctual and arrived almost an hour early. Outside the house he ran into Anna, who directed him to a beautiful backyard garden where he could wait comfortably. At four o'clock, a maid took him up some stairs to a porch.

> At the far end on a couch, dressed in his usual pepper-and-salt suit, lay Professor Freud. He held out his hand but did not rise. "How are you?" he said, and then asked about Margaret. He motioned me to draw my chair nearer. He seemed very frail but keen and alert. After an exchange of the amenities, he said, "I shall not see you today for a regular appointment. To be frank, I am not feeling well. My doctor says my heart is not strong. It's nothing; but he says I had best not work today."[38]

Blanton was concerned and asked whether perhaps he should leave. But Freud assured him that he had no difficulty speaking and inquired about his plans. He had two weeks, maybe a little longer, Blanton replied, the equivalent of twelve sessions. He added that he remembered Freud's preference for dollars and had brought the entire sum for his analysis, a total of $300, in 100-dollar bills. As before, Freud took the money only with the admonition that should he die before the two weeks were up, Blanton must ask to get it back. Freud commented that Blanton had not changed much in three years; Blanton pointed out that it had been five, not three, years since he left Vienna. They talked about recent events.

> "Much water has passed under the bridge, and not all of it clear," I commented. "Ah, yes," he agreed, with a weary shrug. Then he asked how it went with me. I replied that I remained well despite five years of strenuous work, that I hoped I was wiser, and, I continued, "I am happier since my analysis." "Did it help you *personally?*" he asked. "Yes," I replied, "I think it was the most helpful thing—as far as personal understanding—that ever happened to me." He impulsively held out his hand, which I grasped. It was a genuine show of feeling on his part, unusual and spontaneous. "I think of you often and with the deepest affection," I continued.[39]

They agreed to meet two days later, on a Monday, at eleven o'clock. When Blanton arrived for his appointment, he found Freud's physical condition much improved. He lay down on the couch and, after complimenting Freud on his resilience, inquired whether the fee was still $25 as it had been the previous time, an assumption he perhaps should not have made the day before when paying him. Of course, he would make up for the difference should the fee have gone up, he added. Freud waved his concern aside and then asked whether he could afford the $300. If necessary, Freud seemed to be saying, he would gladly see him for less. Blanton answered that he had expected to pay this amount and had set the money aside, even though it required some sacrifices. After this matter was settled, he told Freud that he wanted to speak first about his career, then about his personal life. With Freud's consent, Blanton discussed the politics of the New York Psychoanalytic Institute, his opinion about various colleagues, and the case of a former analytic patient who had killed a woman. Other than expressing his support of Brill, Freud said nothing. Blanton became more aware this time of some of the changes in Freud. He had greater difficulty hearing now, and his speech was unclear, owing to the prosthesis of the jaw and the low voice in which he was speaking. But his presence remained the same.

> Again one is impressed by Freud's ability to be aloof yet at the same time gracious and warm and friendly. His expression of agreement by an indefinite exclamation gives the patient the impression that he is being listened to with great attention (which is the case) and that what he says is important and in agreement with the professor's views. He has learned the difficult art of the countertransference. He gives of himself—but not indiscriminately or in a way that would burden the patient with the necessity of returning affection for affection, of like for like.[40]

In the next meeting Blanton continued talking about work related matters, his colleagues, and patients. Freud said of one of Ferenczi's pupils that she had had a bad influence on him; of Karen Horney he said, "She is able but malicious—mean."[41] He also agreed with Blanton's comment that "an overt homosexual would not make a good analyst."[42] Blanton then brought up the case of a female patient and asked Freud's opinion about her. But Freud said nothing. It was not until Blanton broached a more general theoretical subject, related to women's fantasies about having a penis, that Freud responded. About Blanton's attempt to get him to give advice on his cases, Freud finally said:

> It seems as though you wish to have me work with you as though I were controlling you in your analysis. In a control, you start in the first week and get your impression of the patient—and the next week, and so on. But to enter into a case which has been going on for so long, and whose history is so involved, is impossible. You cannot get an adequate opinion.[43]

But Blanton was not easily deterred and told Freud several of the patient's dreams. Freud again did not comment on the clinical material but answered a general question about how to work with dreams. He also told Blanton that he seemed to be working too hard at making things happen with his patients and that he should concentrate on his technique rather than press for results. In the third hour Blanton brought in some dreams of his own. When Ferenczi came up in his associations, he asked Freud about that analyst's so-called new method. One could understand Ferenczi's technical innovations, Freud said, only in the context of his personal background, at the center of which were early experiences of emotional deprivation.

> "He was one of eleven children. . . . He was starved for love. That was his secret, which came out when he was being analyzed by me. . . . His 'new method'—it had nothing to do with his active therapy, which, by the way, worked very well—was really a passive surrender to the patient. His idea was to satisfy the infantile wishes of the patient. . . . Ferenczi tried to play the part of an overtender father, to give the love he himself had not received and to get love from his patients. That was his secret."[44]

Blanton asked Freud whether he would permit a patient to sit up during an analytic hour or apply makeup or do other such things. Freud answered that he would not allow it and that he would tell the patient, "You are putting yourself out of the analytic situation."[45] After Blanton had given his associations to the dream, Freud made an interpretation that concerned their previous work together: "I get the impression that you were disappointed and dissatisfied, that you wanted to leave before your time, that you wanted to be a member of my family."[46]

Analyst and analysand talked about the technique of dream analysis in general. Freud spoke also, in response to a question, about his three sons, all of whom had to leave Germany because they were Jews. In the following hour Blanton brought in another dream of which he could not make sense and the details of which he does not describe in his journal. Freud said:

> "You seem to be holding back something. . . . It is better not to prepare what you are to say. Come in a more passive attitude." He added that there was something different in my voice; he could not understand me so well. Also, I covered my eyes, and he wondered what this meant. I explained that my eyes hurt me. He also questioned my looking at my watch so often last time. Perhaps it meant that I was bored or that I felt he was not giving me a full hour. On the contrary, I told him, the last hour was most interesting, but my watch had stopped just forty minutes after the hour.[47]

Freud accepted these explanations, saying that they showed how difficult it was to make an interpretation without knowing the patient's associations. However, he later pointed out how Blanton's resistance was manifest in the dream. The university chancellor in the dream represented Freud, Freud said, and Blanton's conscious wish that the chancellor live was an unconscious reversal of the opposite—the wish that he would die.

Blanton reluctantly confessed that he had an idea concerning the nature of his resistance. He wanted Freud to give him permission to include some of their conversations in the autobiography he was planning to write at age 65. Freud wondered why this request embarrassed him; moreover, he was surprised that Blanton wanted to wait until age 65 to write his autobiography.

> [Blanton replied,] "So many people who have known you (like Wittels, for example) have made—I can't think of the word." "Made a mess," Freud interpolated. "Yes," I said, "but that is not the word." Finally it came to me: "Made capital out of you." "Ah," he said, but then repeated, "but you are free to write what you like."[48]

The next day Blanton arrived early and, as he had done previously, waited for his appointment in the garden. This time he found Freud's wife there, busy with a household chore. She was friendly but shy and responded to Blanton's attempt to strike up a conversation with only a smile. The maid came to get him several minutes early, from which gesture Blanton concluded that Freud was trying to spare his wife the embarrassment of the situation. Blanton decided that in the future he would arrive at Freud's house exactly on time. He had brought several new dreams to this analytic hour. Freud commented that this was a sign of resistance since they were not through analyzing the old one. He then suggested that Blanton select the dream that stood out. The associations to the dream, which was about a furry animal, brought up memories of Freud's and Anna's dogs. During the session there was a knock at the door and the chow barked; Freud pointed out with pride what a good watchdog she was. Blanton recalled at this point that one day during his previous analysis he had asked that the dog stay outside during his hour. Freud asked which dog it had been and seemed glad to hear that it had been Anna's dog, Wolf, rather than his, who had caused disturbance— "as though it was a slur on his dog to say she interfered with the analysis."[49] Unlike Wolf, Freud's dog was usually very well mannered and quiet.

Associations to the dream led to a discussion about literature, Robert Graves, and the mental conditions of Caligula and Claudius. Blanton had more questions about technique. He asked whether it was advisable to see a new patient for several trial hours before beginning with the analysis proper; only in the case of a training analysis should this be considered, Freud replied, not with a regular patient. Despite Freud's earlier statement that he could not help him with his clinical cases, Blanton again asked his opinion about a patient. This particular man liked wearing women's underwear, which Blanton attributed to an identification with the mother vis-à-vis the father. Freud agreed but added that it was possible that the patient had not yet achieved true sexual identity; he advised caution when interpreting his fantasies.

In the following hour Blanton continued discussing this particular patient, as well as homosexuality in general. Freud, who seemed bored, spoke of homosexuality as a defense against incestuous impulses toward the mother. Blanton was not sure whether his own somber mood was responsible for Freud's attitude or whether Freud was tired. He discussed another patient. Freud listened but did not say much. At the end of the hour Blanton mentioned that he had once won a bet with his knowledge of the Bible. At issue was Ruth's statement "Entreat me not to leave thee"; to whom had it been addressed? Blanton claimed it was said to Ruth's mother-in-law, but Freud insisted that she had spoken these words to her husband. When they were unable to settle the dispute, Freud promised to check on it.

More than a week had passed in this analysis. The next day Blanton asked Freud to elaborate on a footnote he had found in *The Interpretation of Dreams* that implied a revision of his views on anxiety. Freud referred him to a chapter in the *New Introductory Lectures*. Following this, Blanton gave Freud a lengthy summary of the results from his research on stuttering: He had been able to identify two types of stutterers and reported that several cases involved psychological mechanisms such as oral eroticism, homosexuality, and castration anxiety. Freud, it seemed, was not impressed. He mentioned a case that supported one aspect of Blanton's hypothesis but thought that the symptom was overdetermined and that generalizations about its origin were therefore difficult to make.

Blanton arrived for his next appointment feeling sick. He thought that he had probably contracted a sinus infection, but Freud suggested two possible interpretations: a psychological reaction or a physical response to the climate. Blanton remembered a dream from the preceding night. Queen Victoria is in the company of the Prince of Wales, but she cannot hear him. Whether this is due to her deafness or his poor pronunciation is unclear, but he tells her that despite her difficulty hearing, she is still, unequivocally, ruler of her kingdom. Freud thought it was quite funny that he made an appearance in Blanton's dream as Queen Victoria. He agreed that his hearing was impaired but added that if Blanton would speak more slowly and louder, he could understand everything. The rest of the dream yielded few associations, and Freud commented, "There is still some secret which we have not yet reached."[50] It was not until the following day that Blanton made the connection between the Queen and his own grandmother, which made him the Prince of Wales in the dream. Since Blanton had been raised by his grandmother, the Queen was simultaneously his mother. These associations led to a discussion about homosexuality and the link between Freud, whom Blanton had made a woman in the dream, and his grandmother. When the subject of technique came up again, Freud repeated that he thought Blanton was trying too hard in his clinical work, "Let them work out their own salvation."[51]

The two weeks Blanton had set aside for the analysis were quickly coming to a close. By now Freud was making some suggestions about Blanton's patients; for example, he said that the homosexual aspect of the relationship of one female patient to her mother needed to be explored and would shed light on her attachment to her father. Blanton spoke about the strong women in his life—his mother and grandmother, both determined and hardworking. One of the characteristics his grandmother and Freud shared, Blanton now mentioned, was their stubbornness. He thought Freud was stubborn because he refused to come to the United States for treatment of his dental problems. But Freud replied that he had had a bad experience with the dean of Harvard's dental school. His extensive work on Freud's prosthesis, which cost $6,000, had produced none of the desired results. Blanton thought that the price was exorbitant; he did not believe that this man was the expert he had made himself out to be. He then spoke of Jews and anti-Semitism. He said that the two most brilliant men of the time were both Jewish—Freud and Einstein.

Later in the hour Blanton returned to a subject on which he and Freud disagreed, namely, the United States. On an earlier occasion Freud had been critical of the country, referring to the poor quality of its educational system and culture. "I cannot quote him exactly," wrote Blanton, "but as nearly as I can remember, he had said, 'You Americans are like this: Garlic's good, chocolate's good—let's put a little garlic on chocolate and eat it.' "[52]

Blanton protested Freud's criticisms and tried to convince him of the advantages of living in the United States, advantages such as social equality and freedom. America would eventually prove a fertile ground for the spreading of psychoanalysis, Blanton argued. But Freud was not convinced. He replied that he would like to believe this except that rather the opposite seemed to be true, namely, that psychoanalytic principles were being abused there. For a while Blanton argued his point; then he wondered aloud why he was even talking about this. Freud answered, "It seems to be a sort of exhibitionism."[53] Despite this interpretation, Blanton continued praising his country for its achievements in the social realm. Even in the area of democracy the United States had no more to offer than England did, Freud said. At the end of the analytic hour Blanton felt embarrassed about having shown off. Freud supported his observation that he had bragged in front of him in a childish kind of way but added, "I am sure there must be some deeper reason."[54]

Blanton's last appointment with Freud had arrived. He remembered to return the umbrella the maid had loaned him the day before for the way home. As usual, Freud waited for him in the middle of the room and shook his hand. Blanton asked Freud if he would sign a copy of *The Interpretation of Dreams*, which Freud was happy to do. He then interpreted three dreams, all of which expressed Blanton's wish to be loved by Freud and his desire to stay. Then Blanton proceeded to sum up the results of their work:

> "I seem to have no fundamental neurosis and no fundamental defect that will keep me from practicing analysis successfully." He made an exclamation that gave assent. Then I continued, "I did not get what I expected, which was advice about analysis and patients. But I got something better—a better knowledge of myself and a help in analyzing dreams." Again the professor made an assenting sound.[55]

At the end of the hour Blanton said that he was hoping to be able to return to Vienna the following summer. Freud replied, "I am sorry that I cannot promise to wait for you."[56] After some more amenities they shook hands and Blanton left. As he was walking down the street, he saw Freud standing at the window. Freud waved, then disappeared.

A SECOND RESUMPTION

As it turned out, Blanton did not make it back to Vienna the next year. But in 1937 he and his wife went to Lourdes to study the miracle cures from a medical and psychological point of view. Blanton decided that he, being so close to Vienna, would try to spend another two weeks with Freud. Freud, who was back in Grinzing for the summer with his family, had time to see him; they resumed the analysis on the last day of July. Blanton was now 55, Freud 81.

Blanton arrived half an hour early for his appointment. He waited at the station for a while, then walked slowly toward the house, where he happened upon Freud's daughter and wife. At six o'clock the maid took him into the house. Freud met him in the hallway and commented that he looked well. They entered the consulting room, and Blanton sat down on the couch and discussed his plans. When Freud heard that his wife was with him, he said that he would like to see her. Lying down on the couch, Blanton spoke about his career; he was successful in his private practice, a fact he attributed in part to Freud's help. Then, in answer to a question, he explained that he had come to see Freud for "no special reason, except for the general help you can give and the joy that the hours bring to me."[57]

Blanton said that he and his wife were on their way to Lourdes, and he described the work they were hoping to accomplish there. Freud wanted to know whether he was Catholic (he was not). When Blanton spoke of the claim that Pott's disease had been cured in those shrines, Freud said, "I don't believe it."[58] There were doctors on site who had confirmed this, Blanton argued, and surely they would not all lie. Before long, he gained the impression not only that Freud was unconvinced but that he was not interested in the project. When Blanton drew a parallel to Bernheim's hypnosis cases, Freud made it clear that there was an important distinction. Bernheim's cases were genuine; he himself had witnessed some of them.

For the remainder of the hour, Blanton spoke of a variety of other topics, including research on animals, his analytic cases, and the latest gossip from the New York Psychoanalytic Institute. Freud listened with interest but said little. At one point Blanton mentioned that a friend from the Institute had asked him to get Freud's autograph for him; silence was Freud's only answer. Blanton said that he had heard from someone that Freud did not think well of him as an analyst; Freud replied that it was nothing but a rumor. At the end of the session they discussed appointment times. Blanton preferred noon, and Freud promised to see whether he could arrange for that by trying to change the appointments of the patient he was currently seeing at that hour.

To Blanton, Freud did not seem to have changed much: "He appears to be even more energetic and alert than when I saw him two years ago. He seems very frail, but his movements are as quick as ever. And it was clear that his mind has lost none of its skill and cunning. His hearing seems slightly impaired but no worse than two years ago."[59]

If Blanton talked about personal matters in the next few treatment hours, he did not mention it in his journal. The time for his appointments could not be settled because the patient Freud was going to ask for the change was ill. In his second hour Blanton had some questions regarding wish fulfillment in dreams, which Freud answered. Before the third appointment, Anna called Blanton to change his time from noon to four o'clock. Before lying down on the couch for his third session, Blanton asked Freud whether he could refer him to a dermatologist (he had developed a rash before embarking on his trip to Europe). Freud gave him a name. His wife, Blanton now mentioned, had made him promise to bring up the following question: Should she go to Paris for the two weeks so as not to interfere with the transference? Freud answered, "I could not say yes, and I could not say no."[60] When Blanton mentioned McChord in some context, Freud showed him the bronze head McChord had made of him; it did not look much like him, Freud thought. Blanton told Freud that he did not seem to have changed at all since their first meeting seven years before; Freud was pleased by the compliment but insisted that his hearing had deteriorated further.

The next day Blanton brought in an article he had mentioned earlier about experimental neuroses in sheep. "Freud glanced at it. 'About sheep,' he said and laid the paper on his table."[61] When Blanton gave him another article on spiritual matters, Freud again just said, "About spirits," and put it aside.[62] He asked Blanton whether he had consulted with the dermatologist yet; his appointment was not until later that day, Blanton replied. Blanton then talked about several analysts with whom they were both acquainted. Monroe Meyer, whom Freud had analyzed, had passed on a story about Freud from another American patient, a story Blanton now repeated to Freud. This man claimed that Freud had fallen asleep during one of his analytic hours, owing perhaps, the former patient thought, to his speaking German so poorly.

> During analysis, he heard the professor breathing regularly and deeply. The patient talked louder, but finally he heard the professor let out a little snore. Turning, the patient said, "Professor, you sleep." "*Es macht nichts*" was the reply. ("It doesn't matter.") When I had finished, Freud said, "It is not true. I never slept in my life in an analytical hour. . . . And if the man's German had not been good, I should have told him so." Later, I spoke of working ten hours a day and this being too much. "Well," said Freud, "I did it for many years . . . of course, not now."[63]

Freud returned the article on psychic research the following day. He was not impressed. The study of psychic phenomena, as opposed to telepathy, he argued, would be difficult and time-consuming and, therefore, not worthwhile. In this context Blanton repeated his wish to study the nature of the miracles at Lourdes. But if he had hoped that Freud would finally give his approval of the project, he was disappointed. Freud said nothing.

Before his analytic hour Blanton had the opportunity to meet Freud's new chow; the one Blanton knew from his previous visits had died. In response to Blanton's sympathetic remark that it was hard to lose a dog, Freud said, "It is very hard."[64] After the hour Blanton wrote in his journal, "One gets a feeling of increased power after these visits with the professor. They seem to cause a heightening of one's attention, and to bring to the surface relationships and new conceptions that had lain dormant before."[65]

The next several hours were uneventful. Blanton had a number of theoretical questions, some of them in relation to his own patients, some more general. Freud noticed that he was carrying *The Interpretation of Dreams* with him. He had it with him all the time, Blanton said, and reread it every year. With only four appointments left, Blanton's wife, Margaret, accompanied him and paid Freud a 20-minute visit. They had met before, in 1929, and Freud now asked her about the projects she was working on.

With three appointments left, Blanton paid Freud the money he owed him for 12 sessions.

> "Is this the last day?" he asked. "No," I said, "I come Friday—that makes twelve times. I just went to the bank today and got the money, so I felt it best to give it to you at this time." With a shrug, as though the money were of no importance, he laid it on the table. "Well," he said, "we left some points to be discovered today."[66]

In the next two meetings Blanton asked several general questions about dreams, all of which Freud answered; they also discussed aspects of the oedipal situation and the scientific foundation of faith.

Blanton was sad on his last day. He mentioned it to Freud, but then immediately changed the topic to matters of technique in dream interpretation. At the end of the hour, Blanton said:

> "I should like to come back again." "If I am here, you may," he replied. He then came out into the hall and turned to the porch, while I went out the other end of the hall. As I went through the gate to the street and started down the hill, I looked at his study window. Freud was standing by the window, as on a former time, and waved me good-bye. I raised my hat, then went down the hill and to the car.[67]

A FINAL MEETING

Blanton managed to visit Freud one more time. It was now 1938; Hitler had invaded Austria. Upon urgent entreaties from friends worried about his safety, Freud had finally agreed to move to London. After he was settled there, he received a letter from Blanton, who wanted to study with him for another two weeks. Owing to his health problems, Freud was initially unable to give a definite answer. Toward the end of the summer, however, he wrote a letter to Blanton saying that he had recuperated sufficiently to meet with him in September.

Blanton and his wife arrived in London at the end of August. He called Freud's house immediately and, after several messages, talked to Anna, who scheduled him for five o'clock the following day. Freud was now entering what would be the last year of his life. Yet Blanton's first impression was that Freud appeared much the same. Blanton wrote in his journal, "He seemed as full of energy, as eager and as keen as I had ever seen him."[68] The analysand began the analytic hour by expressing his sympathy with Freud's difficult situation. Freud replied that he considered himself fortunate for having been able to leave at all, thanks to the help of the American government. He and his family were safe, and so was his art collection. He had, however, lost all his money. It was true, he said, that Marie Bonaparte had to pay off the Austrian officials to enable him to depart. But they were here to talk about Blanton, not him, Freud concluded. With this reminder Blanton spoke about his work, and Freud inquired about a particular patient they had discussed before.

The conversation turned again to the political situation. Blanton said he did not think Hitler would go to war, considering that he would have to expect the other powerful nations to unite against him. But Freud was not so sure: "You cannot tell what a madman will do."[69] When Blanton mentioned that he had heard Hitler disliked Freud personally, he got this reply: "I don't know . . . but I hope so."[70] It was painful for him, Freud continued, not to be able to help his Jewish friends in Austria: "You know . . . we are quite helpless to do anything for them."[71] At one point during the hour, Freud had to leave the room owing to the demands of an enlarged prostate. But other than that, he seemed unchanged.

> The overall impression I get of Freud is one of keenness, cheerfulness, alertness, and even gaiety. Perhaps the universal regard which has been shown him in England, as well as the support . . . in Austria, has stirred his spirit. When I said there was also widespread regard for him by people in the United States, he asked, "Do they seem more friendly to me and psychoanalysis?" I assured him of this.[72]

Blanton spent the entire following session analyzing his dreams. He had brought up one dream at the end of the previous hour but had not made much progress with it. By contrast, he was able to understand the meaning of the most recent ones now: They spoke to his wish for more closeness to Freud as well as a feeling of superiority over him; he could also see in them a wish to be young again. Freud said to Blanton, "You are like a boy again in your rejuvenation desires."[73] Later in the hour Blanton asked Freud whether the help he had received from the American government had made him change his low opinion of the United States. No, answered Freud. Blanton repeated his earlier theory that the United States was going to be a good place for psychoanalysis in the future. When Freud did not respond, Blanton spoke in greater detail about his work. After a while he returned to a topic he knew Freud regarded with skepticism, namely, the miracles at Lourdes. He explained that he thought an idealizing mother transference was involved in bringing about the cures. Freud replied that that might be possible. A discussion about technical matters involved in dream work and another unsuccessful attempt on Blanton's part to analyze his earlier dreams brought this hour to a close.

At the next analytic hour Freud asked Blanton whether he had any more associations to the dream of the day before. No, Blanton replied, but he had several new dreams he wanted to work on. They proceeded with the analysis, which was disrupted by much resistance. When their efforts revealed only a general trend in Blanton's unconscious, Freud commented, "You seem to be afraid of something."[74] At the end of the hour they talked more about Freud's new life in England. Freud mentioned that because the new house he had bought was not ready for him to move into, his entire household had to transfer temporarily from this rented house to an émigré hotel.

Analyst and analysand met there the next day. Blanton reminded Freud of his observation in their previous session, that is, that Blanton seemed to be hiding something. He then told Freud that he had avoided bringing up a topic that preoccupied him a great deal—his desire to found a psychoanalytic society in Nashville, Tennessee, after his retirement. What kind of a town was Nashville? Freud inquired. Having learned more details, he seemed to approve. But it was another part of the plan that was now making Blanton nervous. To proceed with it, he needed to become a training analyst first, and he wanted to ask Freud for a letter of recommendation to the New York Psychoanalytic Society. That particular group, Freud answered with bitterness, was currently contemplating a secession from the international group; hence, he had no influence on it whatsoever. In that case, Blanton replied, he would be content to hear Freud's opinion on whether he was a competent analyst and sufficiently capable to be a training analyst. Freud answered in the affirmative.

In the following hour, their fifth meeting, Blanton asked whether Freud's theory of parapraxes allowed for any accidents at all. For instance, should unconscious meaning be attributed to breaking a cup? Freud replied that one might break a cup by accident but slips of the tongue were quite another matter. Blanton eventually returned to the subject of the New York group, admitting that he felt like an outsider. When the hour was almost up, Freud announced that he would have to undergo another surgical procedure on his mouth and would therefore be unable to see him for several days. Blanton was worried, but Freud assured him that he had a good surgeon and would not be in too much pain. He added, with resignation, that this was going to be the 22nd operation in 15 years.

When they met for the next analytic hour, Blanton was reading Bunyan's *Pilgrim's Progress* and talked to Freud about the book, which he considered a work of genius. It seemed odd to Blanton that someone like Bunyan, who was essentially uneducated, could write such a masterpiece. Freud pointed out that being a genius did not necessarily require education and then acknowledged that psychoanalysis was somewhat at a loss when it came to accounting for such extraordinarily gifted people. In reference to Bunyan's book, Blanton discussed the sensitivity with which the subject of death was treated. He thought of what Freud had said about dying. Freud replied, "When you are my age . . . you think of death naturally. But those who think and speak of death are the ones who are not afraid of it. Those who will not speak or think of death are the ones who are afraid of it."[75]

Freud's upcoming operation concerned him, Blanton said. It worried him that he might develop pneumonia again. After Freud had reassured him, Blanton went on to say, "I feel that a lot of the benefit of psychoanalysis is due to the character of the analyst. . . . I think a great deal of the benefit I have had from my analysis is the association with you and the appreciation of your courage, your scientific manner, and your sympathy."[76] Freud did not reply.

The following day Freud informed Blanton that the surgery had been postponed for a couple of days because it had become apparent that it would be more extensive than originally thought; consequently, a longer hospital stay was required. Since Blanton was leaving on September 14 and this was September 6, the next day would be their last meeting. Even though his visit had turned out to be shorter than anticipated, Blanton said, he still felt it had been worthwhile. He added that he was hoping to return the following year for a longer period of time. But Freud answered, "I am afraid I shall not be here."[77] The notes do not reveal whether Blanton said anything about being disappointed that his analysis was coming to such a sudden end. He did, however, speak about his anger toward Freud for not accepting his ideas concerning the case of a boy who was healed in Lourdes, but Freud did not get involved in the argument. When Blanton was ready to leave, Freud reminded him to bring his wife to his last appointment.

Margaret spent the first 10 minutes of her husband's last analytic hour alone with Freud. When Blanton went in, he found Freud in good spirits. He had mentioned before that Freud's positive attitude surprised him. Freud had answered, "Well, perhaps it is on the surface."[78] Blanton paid his bill, which Freud said would cover one week's worth of hospital costs. If Freud was ever in financial difficulties, Blanton said, he would be more than happy to help. Freud graciously declined. The analysis of three recent dreams revealed Blanton's wish that Freud would make a good recovery from his operation and brought up the subject of homosexuality. Freud commented briefly on the wish fulfillment aspect of the first dream and, more generally, on the great resistance in men caused by the thought of homosexual contact. The subject then turned to lay analysis and the differences between the English and American psychoanalytic groups. Freud still did not have much confidence in the Americans but said, "Well, maybe you are the one who may advance the science of psychoanalysis."[79] Blanton told Freud that what he had learned from him as a person was as important as what he had learned from his interpretations and theories and that he deplored the lack of a philosophy that would help men in their 50s and 60s feel content. The end of the hour had come.

> As I finally moved to go, Freud slapped his hand into mine and said, "I should be glad to see you, if I am able, any time you come. . . . Good-bye!" How different this scene of parting, at the Esplanade Hotel, from the two partings before in the old wine village of Grinzing! Since I had seen Freud the year before, the whole world had turned over.[80]

Freud's Treatment Structure

T HE case material in the preceding chapters is rich, compelling, and radically divergent not only from the governing ideals of mainstream technique but even from those guiding the newer analytic approaches. Comparing one's height with that of an analysand or offering a patient a puppy do not constitute either standard or reformed analytic procedure; scolding patients, criticizing their characters, and enjoying correspondence and visits from analysands' friends, spouses, and relatives would be censured by almost any modern analytic school. Reading these cases, one wants to ask: What was Freud doing? Was he simply indulging himself and behaving irresponsibly, or was his conception of treatment different in fundamental ways from our own?

If Freud was practicing psychoanalysis according to different guidelines, we must now identify what these were. Our primary aim in this chapter is to identify Freud's conception of the task of treatment, the method he used to achieve it, and the resulting roles played by the analysis of the transference, the handling of resistances, and the maintenance of neutrality and abstinence. In the interest of gaining a better understanding of these underlying principles, we will of necessity have to sacrifice discussion of the details of each patient's personality and psychopathology, intriguing as these may be. Our second aim in this chapter is to compare Freud's treatment structure to the guidelines he adumbrated in his technique papers, as summarized in Chapter 1, to clarify what contradictions existed between his theory of technique and his behavior in practice.

Even a cursory reading of the material just presented shows that neutrality and the analysis of transference did not play central roles in

Freud's clinical work, as they do in analytic practice today. Further, it is apparent that Freud's understanding of resistance analysis was different from our own. We shall see, however, that these differences are not due to a lack of technique, as has been suggested. Rather, they are the result of the way Freud defined the primary task of the treatment and the structure he created in order to achieve it—namely, making the unconscious conscious and employing the "technology" of free association in the division of labor between himself and his patient. Dreams, analyzed by free association, were of great significance as well inasmuch as Freud considered dreams the most direct and accessible derivatives of the unconscious. Freud's definition of the analytic task and the centrality of free association as the means of accomplishing it determined the place of other aspects of procedure.

THE PRIMARY TASK:
MAKING THE UNCONSCIOUS CONSCIOUS

In her account of her treatment with Freud, H.D. described an instance when he suddenly seemed angry; he was beating with his fist on the head-piece of the couch, charging that she did not think it worth her while to love him because he was an old man. She added to her description: "And even as I veered around, facing him, my mind was detached enough to wonder if this was some idea of *his* for speeding up the analytic content or redirecting the flow of associated images."[1] It is clear that H.D. habitually made use of withdrawal and intellectualization in defense against difficult personal situations, but her suggestion here that Freud's seemingly emotional outburst was also quite purposefully aimed at advancing their work captures an element in his technique noted by many other of his patients.

Joan Riviere, for instance, a British analyst and future Kleinian who was analyzed by Freud in 1922 and later translated some of his papers into English (Jones, 1959), described Freud's interest and enthusiasm during her analysis as "curiously impersonal. One had always the impression of a certain reserve behind the eagerness, as though it were not for himself that he so peremptorily demanded to understand things, but for some purpose outside himself."[2] This "purpose outside himself" was the primary task, or goal, of the treatment: to bring to light the patient's unconscious wishes, thoughts, conflicts, and memories. Freud told Wortis, "The psychoanalytic cure consists in bringing unconscious material to consciousness."[3]

Making the unconscious conscious could theoretically refer to unconscious aspects of the ego, such as defenses, which Freud knew (and had known for decades by the time he treated the patients presented in this book) were central in the formation of neuroses; these would manifest as resistance to the treatment. But Freud's interpretations in these patients' accounts of their analyses show clearly that even at this late point in his career the primary object of his interest was the unconscious content, not the process by which it remained repressed or hidden from consciousness.

Freud's definition of the primary task meant getting to the bottom of things, discovering what secrets motivated patients without their conscious knowledge. Freud had a passion for finding the truth behind the symptoms and symbols, a passion that was reflected in, among other things, the many interpretations that would now be considered "deep" and that even Freud, according to his writings on technique, would have considered so. In fact, a number of his comments and interventions, as well as his patients' descriptions of them, were quite literally concerned with "depth." Recall H.D.'s experience of Freud's eagerness to get to the root of her resistance—"Papa is drilling away like mad this time;"[4] his satisfaction when telling her, "Today we have tunneled very deep;"[5] and his observation when they were discussing the Van Eck episode that they had "gone into deep matters."[6] He consoled Blanton that he needed to be patient, promising, "We will get to the deeper layers"[7]; on another occasion he told him, "There is still some secret we have not yet reached."[8] Kardiner expressed the same idea when he pleaded with Freud in a dream to stop "digging."[9] And, in a conversation with H.D., Freud likened his discovery of psychoanalysis to striking oil.[10]

Defining the task as making the unconscious conscious is in accordance with Freud's theoretical view of the aim of psychoanalytic treatment in the broadest sense. Consider the following two sections from *An Outline of Psycho-Analysis* (1940a), in which Freud described the "plan of cure" as consisting of strengthening the ego and weakening the power and influence of id and superego:

> The ego is weakened by the internal conflict and we must go to its help. The position is like that in a civil war which has to be decided by the assistance of an ally from outside. The analytic physician and the patient's weakened ego, basing themselves on the real external world, have to band themselves together in a party against the enemies, the instinctual demands of the id and the conscientious demands of the super-ego.[11]

This is accomplished in the following way:

> The sick ego promises us the most complete candour . . . we assure the patient of the strictest discretion and place at his service our experi-

ence in interpreting material that has been influenced by the unconscious. Our knowledge is to make up for his ignorance and to give his
ego back its mastery over lost provinces of his mental life.[12]

In other words, the task is to strengthen the ego by bringing to light
unconscious material; here Freud's stated aim is very much in keeping
with what we have seen in the cases. In fact, this conceptualization of
how the ego will regain control is reflected in some literal and derivative
allusions to light—the corollary to the depth metaphor—in the clinical
data. On one occasion, for example, Freud showed Money-Kyrle (an
English psychologist who had been analyzed by Jones previously and later
became a Kleinian) "his Euchaptis to explain that their colour was fading
because they had been dug up—like relics from the unconscious."[13] In
another instance Freud asked H.D. whether her memories were "faded."[14]
Knowledge equals light. His patients, too, conjured up images of light
when describing Freud and his insights with words such as "brilliant" and
"illuminating." H.D. wrote Bryher triumphantly that they might be
contributing to the development of analytic theory: "Perhaps you and I
. . . ARE to be instrumental in some way in feeding the light." Freud's use
of metaphors such as depth, light, and layers shows his continued alle-
giance to the topographical model, in which the psyche is pictured as
layered consciousness.[15]

It can be said, then, that there is agreement between Freud's theory
of the analytic task and his clinical behavior: Making the unconscious
conscious was the aim of the treatment, and Freud's mode of work reflects
this. In terms of his procedural suggestions on how to get there, however,
the matter is more complicated. As we discussed in Chapter 1 with regard
to interpretation, Freud vacillated throughout his technical writings between two positions, which were never reconciled. In one approach the
analyst makes interpretations of repressed, unconscious content before the
patient is ready to discover it for himself—"to create an impression . . . so
that it may work upon him."[16] For instance, in the section from *An Outline
of Psycho-Analysis* quoted earlier, Freud goes on to say that the patient

> will present us with a mass of material—thoughts, ideas, recollec-
> tions—which are already subject to the influence of the unconscious,
> which are often its direct derivatives, and which thus put us in a
> position to conjecture his repressed unconscious material and to
> extend, by the information we give him, his ego's knowledge of his
> unconscious.[17]

In the other approach the analyst works with the ego and its resistances,
that is, works only with what the patient presents him or her, works from

the surface down, and refrains from taking an "intellectualist" view of the situation.

In the clinical data there are very few instances of Freud working from the surface down; many of his interpretations show that he continued to regard resistance as an obstacle to uncovering unconscious contents, an obstacle that needed to be removed in the pursuit of the task. A much-criticized example of this procedure can be found in his treatment of the Rat Man, a case in which Freud guessed that the anus was the body part involved in the cruel rat torture rather than analyzing Lorenz's resistance to naming it. When H.D. was in the middle of a story about a piece of paternal trickery, Freud finished it "before [she] had time to tell him."[18] Apparently, as the father of six, Freud was only too familiar with the little lies parents make up to keep the peace and protect the illusion of their beneficence. Moreover, there was nothing in his conception of treatment that prevented him from actually being paternal at that particular moment while remaining a transference object.

Instances of Freud's passion for unearthing lost memories, for exposing the nucleus of the symptom complex—reminiscent of his search for what he called the *caput Nili,* or origin of neurosis, in the founding days of psychoanalysis—run through all his published cases.[19] How deeply satisfying making such discoveries continued to be for Freud even in or because of advanced age can be gleaned from an incident reported by Alix Strachey: Freud, after the interpretation of a particularly difficult dream, lit a cigar with the words, "Such insights need celebrating."[20] Similarly with H.D., he was "always making an 'occasion' of it, get[ting] up and say[ing], 'Ah—now—we must celebrate *this,*' and proceed[ing] to the elaborate ritual" of selecting and lighting a cigar.[21] Some analysts have referred to this treatment approach as id, rather than ego, psychology, arguing that Freud never put into effect the changes in technique they thought were implied with the formal advent of the structural model of the mind in 1923. We shall have more to say about this and the matter of resistance analysis later.

Freud wrote that to accomplish the task of making the unconscious conscious the analyst forms an alliance with the patient's weakened ego: The patient promises to say whatever comes to mind without censorship, and the analyst interprets the unconscious basis of that material. Nonetheless, Freud's clinical work shows that he still expected the patient to be capable of mobilizing his observing and analyzing functions and to work cooperatively. Freud quarreled with his patients when they were not ready or willing to hear what he had to say. Some of his analysands, like H.D. and Blanton, relished being challenged in this way—most of the time, that is. Others felt that Freud expected too much of them. Adjectives such as "shattered, battered, sick" were used by H.D. to describe her emotional states following some analytic hours, and Kardiner described feeling "agitated, disturbed, bewildered."[22] Maryse Choisy, a French woman from an aristocratic family who later became an analyst herself, fled in a panic following a dream interpretation by Freud that suggested the solution of a longtime family secret; she felt altogether overestimated by Freud: "He believed he could tell me anything. . . . He interpreted too early."[23]

Freud expected his patients to be able to rise above their neurotic symptoms and resistances, to mobilize within themselves the more mature aspects of their personalities, and to hear what was in their unconscious—regardless of their psychopathology. Freud's criticism of Wortis for not being willing to face unpleasant truths about himself illustrates this: "That is not a scientific attitude. . . . You have not yet completed the transition from the pleasure principle to the reality principle."[24] Freud's intervention here is striking not only because he did not analyze Wortis's resistance but also because he treated Wortis's narcissism no differently than Kardiner's neurosis—except with more irritation and impatience. Current theories on the treatment of narcissistic patients stress these individuals' sensitivity to criticism and advocate empathy and "mirroring" as the primary tools of technique. Obviously, Freud and Kohut would have answered the question of what is curative in the psychoanalysis of such patients differently, but what is clear, in any event, is that Freud was not thinking of his patients—regardless of diagnosis—as adults *manqués*, or children masquerading as grown-ups, who need to be parented or coddled into health. On the one hand, it seems that Freud misjudged some of his patients' ability to engage in this kind of work, which relies on a great deal of sacrifice, effort, and active participation on the part of the analysand; on the other hand, this approach allowed for an analytic experience in which important things could be said and discovered by analyst and patient and in which the patient was treated as a person capable of adult work. Later we will have more to say about this, too.

Making the unconscious conscious is, in theory, not specific with respect to content. This was the position Freud originally took when first listening to his patients' free associations. By not assigning an a priori meaning to the material that would emerge, Freud had been able to develop an entire theory of the mind. His approach to treatment retained this empirical research aspect; Dorsey, for instance, commented on the "untendentious nature of his psychoanalytic devotion to observation of what was happening in free association."[25] Freud conveyed to other patients as well a sense of openness as to what might be found. H.D. quite basked in the experience of herself as "this one ego under the microscope-telescope of Sigmund Freud."[26] In another place she commented:

> [T]he Professor said, "there is always more to find out." . . . It was
> almost as if something I had said was *new*, that he even felt that I was
> a *new* experience. He must have thought the same of everyone, but I
> felt his personal delight, I was *new*. Everyone else was *new*, every dream
> and dream association was *new*. After the years and years of patient,
> plodding research, it was all *new*.[27]

Some of his analysands were even aware that they might be contributing to the formulation of new theories. H.D. believed that she and
Bryher had given Freud new ideas about penis envy and other aspects of
the psychology of women,[28] which clearly satisfied her need for special-
ness and may have inspired even greater efforts on her part to make
herself interesting to Freud. And we know how important particular
cases—the Rat Man and the Wolf Man, among others—were for the
development of large pieces of Freud's theory. At times, Freud's preoccupation with the development of new theories could, by his own
admission and the testimony of his patients, get in the way of the
treatment. Some people have said that his interest in theory made him
a less effective clinician. Raymond de Saussure, a Swiss psychoanalyst
in treatment with Freud in the early '20s, concluded that Freud was not
a good "technician. . . . One rapidly sensed what special theoretical
question preoccupied him, for often during the analytic hour he developed at length new points of view he was clarifying in his own mind.
This was a gain for the discipline, but not always for the patient's
treatment."[29]

It was Freud's passion not only for discovering hidden meaning but
also for recognizing the potential of a given case for adding missing pieces
to the theory that appeared to make some analyses more interesting to
him. H.D., who thrived on the colorful, the extraordinary, and even the
occult, and her labyrinthian tale about the mysterious Van Eck and the
"Writing on the Wall" seemed intrinsically more fascinating to Freud
than did the more plodding Dorsey, to whom Freud said little. Freud was
clearly curious, intrigued, and eager to unravel her story and piece
together the bits of memory, poetry, and mysticism into a cogent psychological narrative. Moreover, his way of working allowed him to tell her
that he was curious about how her story would proceed: He rushed out of
the room exclaiming, "I have an idea!" and returned with a leather
suitcase in an effort to trace the origin of Van Eck's name; he said that
the Corfu experience had made him think "very hard."[30]

While Freud had started out his career knowing very little about
what he might find in his patients' unconscious, he obviously had a better
idea as time went on and was not perfectly "untendentious," as Dorsey
would have it. Kardiner pointed out that Freud's method and interpreta-

tions in general were simple and unencumbered by theoretical assumptions, his focus on the Oedipus complex, with attendant death wishes and unconscious homosexuality, being the main exceptions. While interpretations of the Oedipus complex, unconscious homosexuality, and the primal scene were part of the standard fare of nearly every analysis, there were interpretations of many other phenomena—for example, penis envy, the girl's preoedipal attachment to the mother, bisexuality, and back-to-the-womb wishes. And there were, of course, case-specific interpretations.

Once a patient's core unconscious dynamics were unearthed, Freud thought the work was, in essence, completed. After he saw from H.D.'s dreams that she had made the connection between the war years and earlier experiences, he declared her analysis more or less over.[31] And toward the end of their second round together, Freud referred to her analysis as finished once she had realized the bisexual core of her conflicts.[32] His patients at times disagreed with his judgment: Kardiner, who did not share Freud's opinion that his treatment was "complete and perfect,"[33] suggested that, in particular, the analysis of the transference was left undone, but Freud apparently was satisfied with the result of their work, which had centered on the analysis of oedipal themes and unconscious homosexuality.

Thus, in summary, there are several important characteristics of the primary task in Freud's technique. It involved bringing to light patients' unconscious conflicts in order to increase their knowledge and control over the lost domains of the ego. When the patient was a student, the treatment had the secondary major task of teaching about psychoanalytic theory and procedure. In the case of neurotics, once the unconscious contents were known and made intelligible to secondary process thinking, the ego was considered strengthened and the patient cured. Therefore, Freud concerned himself only with attending to the task and method as described above and not with effecting therapeutic results beyond the treatment. Making the unconscious conscious *was* the cure. Freud showed his disregard for more distant outcomes in his advice to student analysands to not worry about making their own patients better. Rather, they should help them speak their minds freely. He told Blanton, "You are perhaps too anxious about your patients. . . . You must let them drift. Let them work out their own salvation."[34]

The task in Freud's conception of treatment was well defined, which made therapeutic progress easily measurable, and yet it was theoretically unspecific with regard to content, leaving open the particulars of interpretations and the shape of the analytic relationship that followed. Most importantly, however, Freud had a method—free association—which was well suited for accomplishing the task.

THE METHOD: FREE ASSOCIATION

Freud considered free association the sine qua non for achieving the aim of the treatment; it was the means by which unconscious material could surface and the means by which adherence to the task could be monitored. He actively conveyed to his patients the importance of following the fundamental rule, of exploring their unconscious without judging it in advance from either a theoretical or a moral point of view. Freud was extremely critical of Wortis's preconceived ideas about the meaning of his dreams and associations. He found it rendered their work useless. For similar reasons, recall that he told Blanton not to hold anything back:

> He then repeated the admonition about giving free reign to the unconscious, without reservations. "You are not responsible for your unconscious. . . . While you are bringing up the material, you must not have any moral judgments about it. . . . It is only one step from excusing the material from your unconscious to being insecure in telling what is in the unconscious."[35]

Censorship interfered with free association and the full understanding of the patient's mind; therefore, it had to be avoided.

Freud had realized early that the meaning of symptoms was locked away in his patients' unconscious mind, but only gradually did he discover that he had to let them speak freely to allow it to emerge. The task of making the unconscious conscious and the method of free association were powerfully linked from the start; together they led to the formulation of the fundamentals of psychoanalytic theory. The special fit between the two is due to the fact that, conceptually and phenomenologically, they form a matrix and overlap: When one free-associates, one is performing the task. The relationship between the outcome—uncovering hidden meaning—and the method that will bring it about—giving voice to unbidden thoughts without censorship—is one of intrinsic interdependence. It is the inevitability of this connection that made free association a powerful procedural tool and that explains why Freud could rely on it alone to form the basis of his treatment structure.

The patient's willingness to accept the fundamental rule was key to the success of an analysis. Therefore, Freud instructed new analysands in this method and reminded those with a knowledge of psychoanalysis how they were to proceed. Wortis wrote about his first hour:

> I was directed to a couch. Freud sat behind me and commenced a little lecture on the ensuing procedure, talking in true lecture style, deliberately and lucidly. . . . He then went on to speak of the fundamental

condition for an analysis: absolute honesty—I was to tell literally everything that went through my head: whether important, unimportant, painful, irrelevant, absurd, or insulting.[36]

With most of his patients, Freud had to repeat his instructions more than once. Blanton understood what he was supposed to do but was immediately resistant. Freud told him to relax. When he came in the next day with a prepared account of his childhood, Freud told him not to prepare what he was going to say: "give freely what comes into your mind. That is the classical method."[37] In later hours Freud was encouraging him not to let any fears get in the way of his associations: "It is necessary for the unconscious to express itself freely"; "You must follow the rule of analysis and be free to let your mind go as it will."[38] Freud reminded Wortis, "Anything will do, past or present, since it is all of one piece, and our purpose is to see the structure of your mind, like an anatomist."[39]

For Dorsey, learning how to free-associate became the focus of the entire analysis: "[N]ot withholding speaking of *any* mental content for any reason whatsoever, was my one psychoanalytic rule."[40] He added that Freud was "strict" with respect to his observance of it.[41] When he finally managed to talk without holding back, Freud said, "That is free association."[42]

To gain the most uncensored view of the unconscious, not only was the patient required to free-associate but the work had to be spontaneous in other respects as well. Freud told H.D. several times that she should not prepare for her hours by writing notes or sending daily reports to Bryher with a blow-by-blow account of her treatment. When he realized that Blanton had decided in advance what he was going to say, Freud reminded him, "Come in a more passive attitude."[43] He asked Wortis not to tell his wife about his analysis. However, as with most other rules, Freud was willing to make exceptions. After having told Blanton not to prepare, he let him give the prepared account anyway. While advising H.D. and Marie Bonaparte not to take notes, he did not seem to object to it in the cases of Blanton and Wortis.

As noted, the strength of Freud's conviction about the effectiveness of a treatment based upon free association has its roots in the very beginnings of psychoanalysis. Free association had been at the center of Freud's work since the mid-1890s. Indeed, it seems that he may well have been using the technique, along with other methods, from the beginning of his private practice work in the late 1880s.[44] An important aspect of the history of psychoanalysis concerns the winnowing out of other procedures in favor of an exclusive reliance upon free association, a transition that required some 15 years. Free association not only proved to be valuable therapeutically, it was also the source of analytic knowledge. The method preceded the theory in the history of psychoanalysis and continued to precede theoretical formulations in the treatment of the individual. The empirical orientation in Freud's work remained an important aspect of his technique. Thus, the method of free association was intimately linked not only to the therapeutic task but also to Freud's ongoing research endeavors.

Freud wrote that free association became the "precondition of the whole analytic treatment."[45] Less of a strain on both patient and doctor than earlier techniques had been, it kept the patient in close contact with the actual current situation, and it guaranteed "to a great extent that no factor in the structure of the neurosis [would] be overlooked and that nothing [would] be introduced into it by the expectations of the analyst. It was left to the patient to determine the course of the analysis and the arrangement of the material. . . . Another advantage of the method [was] that it need never break down. It must theoretically always be possible to have an association, provided that no conditions are made as to its character."[46]

After the early years of working arduously at getting his patients to do one particular thing or another, the discovery that free association was not only more useful clinically but also presented less of a strain on the analyst was a welcome one to Freud. Considering the fact that for many years he was seeing ten patients a day for six days a week, the practical advantage of listening "composedly but without any constrained effort to the stream of associations,"[47] rather than forcing connections or events, can easily be appreciated. More importantly, this way of listening ensured a state of mind in the analyst—called free-floating or evenly hovering attention—that made him particularly receptive and attuned to the patient's unconscious. In this new division of labor, the patient gave associations and the analyst responded, usually silently, with counterassociations, a process that eventually led to the formulation of the meaning of the patient's material. Freud thought that the ability to interpret unconscious derivatives was due not to some innate talent or special intuition but, rather, to a state of mind that could be achieved by anyone who was not inhibited by too much resistance.[48] All of Freud's patients attested to the fact that he was brilliantly insightful. Recall Wortis's saying to Freud on one occasion, "Your conclusions are often more convincing than your methods. . . . You seem to have a special kind of incommunicable intuition." "It is not intuition," said Freud, "it is just ready association. You happen not to associate so readily where your unconscious is concerned."[49]

In free association, patients are under the least amount of pressure by the analyst and are left to determine the course of the material themselves. However, this freedom is relative, perhaps not unlike free association itself. Freud noted, "We must, however, bear in mind that free association is not really free. The patient remains under the influence of the analytic situation even though he is not directing his mental activities on to a particular subject."[50] Earlier we gave examples of the way in which Freud repeatedly encouraged his patients to determine the course and content of the analytic hour by speaking freely. However, there are also many examples of Freud's intervening and redirecting the flow of associations through interpretations and other interventions. For example, he told Wortis to talk more about his problems.[51] And he made H.D. talk the whole hour about Ezra Pound.[52] And then, of course, there were the numerous discussions between analyst and patient about art, psychoanalytic theory, and the like, which Freud at times initiated.

The seeming paradox in Freud's behavior can be attributed to several factors. First, the analyst's freedom is also only relative since, like the patient, he or she is under a requirement to perform the task and to conform to a role corresponding to the patient's, namely, to listen with an evenly hovering attention leading to interpretation or other facilitating utterances. When task performance was poor, Freud could thus not allow free association to continue uninterrupted.

Second, the paradox of free association being free yet prescribed as a fundamental *rule* encountering various limits is due to the fact that the pact between analyst and patient is based on "the real external world."[53] Freud's analysands were constantly reminded of the external world in his consulting room by his very real presence. In fact, sometimes the couch itself was not safe from intrusions—with Freud hammering on its head-piece with his fist triumphantly or impatiently. H.D., half complaining, half relieved, wrote Bryher that she was not allowed to just "dream and fantasize." Therefore, not only were patients' associations necessarily bound to the exigencies of the analytic treatment, including the requirement to accomplish the task (that is, discover the unconscious), but the patients themselves were grounded in the reality of a relationship with the analyst.

Free association was in the service of a task; it was a means to an end, not the end itself, and did not constitute the whole of the analytic relationship or technique. If it could be interrupted, it could also be reinstated. H.D. wrote Bryher that Freud was getting stricter about limiting their conversations to topics related to the analysis.[54] From this perspective it can be said that, although Freud's activity constitutes an interference with the patient's self-expression, it also functions (within bounds) as a necessary delimitation. In Freud's technique the task was as important to the relationship and the overall enterprise as intrapsychic structure is to the individual. And structure in Freud's treatment was provided not only by a clear, coherent, and stable division of labor and by his interpretations but also, crucially, by his real and authoritative presence as the leader of the enterprise.

Thus, Freud can be observed responding to his patients' associations with his own ideas; some of these were related to the material whereas others seem to have arisen from his own concerns. At times, Freud's interventions seem to have been merely self-indulgent (such as engaging in gossip or getting into an extended dialogue with the patient about theory) and perhaps reflect his own resistance and rebellion toward the task or his weariness with the unrelenting nature of his obligation to it. Freud called the working through of resistances an "arduous task for the subject of the analysis and a trial of patience for the analyst."[55]

A further way of understanding the relationship between spontaneity and limit, or obligation, is to say that through free association Freud delegated the leadership for the agenda to the patient while he remained present and in charge as the person responsible for the overall enterprise (Newton, 1989). As we have seen, Freud was actively directive about making free association the primary requirement of the patient in the division of analytic labor. His most important tools in this endeavor were his instruction and then encouragement and reminders to the patient to free-associate. He told Blanton, "You must follow the rule of analysis and be free to let your mind go as it will."[56]

Freud kept the primary task in focus by making the state of the treatment enterprise itself a matter for discussion. When things were going well, meaning that the patient was associating without much resistance, Freud expressed his satisfaction. For instance, he told Wortis, "We have moved a little forward,"[57] and "Fine . . . that's what I call real analysis."[58] But a patient whose resistance was interfering with free association heard unequivocally about that, too. Freud told Blanton, "Today has been absolutely sterile."[59] He could be very impatient in such instances; Wortis's stubborn resistance to speak his mind freely not only was a source of annoyance for Freud but was identified by him as one of the key problems in their therapeutic stalemate. Freud told him that he had "too many ideas and too few associations."[60]

Freud did not hesitate to be directive in other ways, when necessary, and to shape the proceedings of the analysis to improve task performance. For instance, he asked Blanton to bring in dreams. When H.D., in his estimation, had talked enough about the war period, he asked her to discuss her early childhood. These examples show Freud keeping a watchful eye on the work and reveal his willingness to intervene, even in free association.

From the aforementioned clinical material, it is clear that free association had a much more central role in Freud's clinical work than it does in analytic work today. Even though it is still considered a valuable tool, only a minority of analysts place their analysands under an explicit requirement to use it. Lichtenberg and Galler (1987) surveyed an international sample of eminent analysts and found that only 37 percent followed Freud's recommendations about instituting free association as the fundamental rule of the treatment. Note that these respondents were eminent analysts, which means that the impact of their views on analytic practice today, through their writing and teaching, is extensive. An important concern expressed by many of these analysts was the possibility that instructing patients or reminding them of what to do might increase their resistance. Lichtenberg and Galler note that from Freud's time to our own, analysts have become less comfortable with the overt use of authority. Newton (1971, 1973a, 1973b, 1989, 1992a) has written at length about the problems attendant upon the clinician's eschewing or disguising his or her authority. This eschewal of rational (that is, limited to that required by the nature of the task) authority is compounded when the clinician construes the task as remedial child rearing and his relationship to the patient as one between grown-up and child. Here, the rational authority between two adults in work is transformed into parental authoritarianism, however gentle its tone and benevolent its purpose.

Since in Freud's view the work of analytic treatment was to make the unconscious conscious through free association, other aspects of technique considered essential by contemporary standards were of lesser significance to him, in particular, those having to do with neutrality and transference analysis, which we will discuss in greater detail later. The reliance upon free association allowed Freud to be spontaneous and real with his patients and to engage in a number of behaviors that would now be called unanalytic by many. As Lipton (1977) pointed out, technique for Freud had a more circumscribed role in the overall relationship and specific behaviors were secondary to the task of the treatment.

Among other things, this meant that Freud was able to use his person and associations much more actively in the work. Joan Riviere commented that "he was so concentrated on the inquiry he was pursuing that his self functioned only as an instrument."[61] As we have seen, Freud was very involved in the treatments of some of his patients; he let them know he was interested in their conflicts, dreams, and thoughts. Recall his exclamation to H.D. that "if he lived another fifty years, he would still be fascinated and curious about the vagaries and variations of the human mind or soul."[62] Riviere, as well, was impressed with Freud's enthusiasm; she described the beginning of their first meeting as follows: " 'Well, [said Freud,] I know something about you already; you had a father and a mother!' meaning of course, 'Quick, I can't wait for you and your inhibitions, I want something to start with.' "[63]

Freud's attitude toward the work helped establish the formation of a strong therapeutic alliance and made the pursuit of the task a collaborative effort, in contrast to the unilaterality in the analytic relationship that came to be accepted in the 1950s with the basic model technique (Lipton, 1977), a development we will discuss shortly. What Freud exemplified for his patients was a commitment to finding the truth, a commitment that was apparent in his general concern with honesty and accuracy and demonstrated concretely by his tendency to consult dictionaries or encyclopedias to ascertain facts. This commitment to truth was, among other things, an example to his patients of how to approach the analytic work as a whole; for example, Freud told Wortis, "I told you unpleasant things about yourself to show you how honest one is in analysis."[64]

DREAM ANALYSIS

When he was approaching termination of his treatment, Dorsey asked Freud what he thought had helped him most in understanding the nature of his problems. Without hesitation Freud referred to a particular dream. The work with dreams played a key role in every treatment inasmuch as dreams represent the most direct derivatives of the unconscious; Freud likened them to neurotic symptoms and psychoses.[65] He had always been fond of dreams and his *Interpretation of Dreams* (1900) became the favorite among his books. In his self-analysis dreams had provided critical evidence regarding important theoretical discoveries, such as the Oedipus complex. It is interesting to note that the first of Freud's papers on technique was about working with dreams, as was his first case study (Dora). Their significance can be understood in terms of their special relationship to task and method; to fathom the meaning of dreams Freud could once again rely on free association.

Affording the most unhampered view into the unconscious, dreams were useful in the analysis of every patient. But they could be especially helpful when the patient was not neurotic or very resistant; then dreams could furnish material to work with or explanations as to what was going on. From Blanton's dreams Freud was able to interpret resistance and negative transference, which appeared only very subtly in their relationship. He told Wortis after 10 days that he had been waiting for him to bring in dreams to see whether enough material would be forthcoming for an analysis. Wortis's dreams, however, were no less affected by resistance than were his associations, and they contributed little by way of insight. When he finally reported a dream that was full of interesting symbols, Freud exclaimed, "That's what I call a real dream."[66] In order not to overlook anything in the patient's mind that would be worth knowing about, Freud insisted on dreams being part of the treatment.

Freud's procedure for dream analysis demanded that the patient first say what came to mind about particular dream elements, engaging in a kind of directed free association. Freud attributed greater significance to these associations than to universal symbols. After Blanton had given his thoughts on one of his dreams, Freud said, "You can never tell what a thing means until you have associated to it."[67] However, there are also many instances in which Freud referred to the inherent meaning of dream symbols, that is, to their inborn and presumably universal character and origin in folklore and philology.[68] There are several examples of this in Wortis's treatment: Freud said that the fish was "a well-known symbol for the penis"; that little animals "always meant females"; that "falling is a constant symbol for femininity, for giving birth or being born"; that "eating is a natural symbol for one's mother"; and that "fleas and insects meant children as a rule."[69] He told Blanton that the car was a "frequent symbol for psychoanalysis."[70]

As with free association, the ideas about a dream can be useless if they are affected by too much resistance. In such instances Freud sometimes argued over an interpretation and, not infrequently, insisted that he was right. Freud's disagreement with Oberndorf about his dream, recounted by Kardiner, is one example.

After the patient had presented his associations, Freud usually added his own. He was brilliant in the interpretation of dreams—even "uncanny,"[71] according to Kardiner. From them he could guess all kinds of secrets and sometimes the entire structure of a neurosis. For instance, he understood the full implications of Kardiner's dreams about the urinating Italians in terms of the Oedipus complex and his transference to Frink. From another dream he discovered that Kardiner had been present when his mother died.

Maryse Choisy, mentioned earlier in this chapter, described her brief experience in psychoanalysis with Freud. In her third session she spoke of a dream, in association with which, by her own admission, not much occurred to her, but Freud was still able to tell her "that such and such event happened when [she was] still in the cradle."[72] She was shocked and returned to France immediately to confront her family. Freud had been right. The event he had divined turned out to be a well-kept family secret to which Choisy had not been made privy (and whose details are not passed on to the reader). She did not resume her treatment: "Freud now symbolized for me the magical father, the medicine-man. He saw through me. I felt as transparent as glass. I was scared."[73] Choisy did not return to psychoanalysis for another eight years.

Similarly, in the third week of his analysis of the Greek Princess Marie Bonaparte, which took place in 1925, Freud inferred from a dream that she had witnessed sexual intercourse as a child. Bonaparte protested, but Freud said that her associations confirmed his impression. Later, with the help of journals she had kept as a young girl, they were able to reconstruct what had happened: At a young age she had indeed watched her nursemaid having an affair with the head groom, Pascal, over an extended period of time. Freud guessed various other details related to this situation, all of which Pascal confirmed upon Bonaparte's return to Paris.[74]

Freud had first come to understand the significance of dreams in his work with neurotics. Indeed, he understood the role of wish fulfillment in dreams earlier than in neurosis, as early as 1895.[75] It was not until two years later that Freud saw that neurotic symptoms, too, involved the fulfillment of a wish; indeed, a fuller understanding of neurosis had to await, and arose directly from, his work on the *The Interpretation of Dreams*.[76] In therapy he came to treat dreams like all other symptoms: The patient had to associate to them. While also subject to distortions from the ego and resistances, dreams still afforded an especially unimpeded view of unconscious conflicts and mechanisms. But to understand them, free association was once again the key.

With the help of the method of free association and of the closely related art of interpretation, psychoanalysis succeeded in achieving something that appeared to be of no practical importance but that led to a "fresh attitude and a fresh scale of values in scientific thought. It became possible to prove that dreams have meanings and to discover them."[77]

Freud had noticed a link between free association and the interpretation of dreams in his work with Emmy von N., whose treatment he described in *Studies on Hysteria*, which he wrote with Breuer in the mid-1890s. After having pointed out the tendency of neurotic patients to bring into connection with each other ideas that were simultaneously present in their minds, Freud stated that he had noticed the same "compulsion towards association" in his dreams.[78] In *The Interpretation of Dreams* Freud gave the following account of how he began to work with dreams:

> My patients were pledged to communicate to me every idea or thought that occurred to them in connection with some particular subject; amongst other things they told me their dreams and so taught me that a dream can be inserted into the psychical chain that has to be traced backwards in the memory from a pathological idea. It was then only a short step to treating the dream itself as a symptom and to applying to dreams the method of interpretation that had been worked out for symptoms.[79]

Thus, dreams had played a key role in Freud's discovery of psychoanalysis and remained a central part of his clinical technique. An especially useful means of accomplishing the task, dreams represented a kind of shortcut to the secrets of the patient's unconscious. The full interpretations Freud gave illustrate the way in which resistances and defenses were bypassed rather than analyzed.

HANDLING OF RESISTANCE

Freud had understood early that resistance lay at the root of his patients' inability to tell him about their unconscious thoughts. Indeed, he complained about his own resistances to his friend Wilhelm Fliess when, during the fall of 1897, he was in the midst of a mid-life crisis (Newton, 1995). Freud had lost hold of the seduction theory and was banking on his self-analysis to lead him to a new solution to the problem of neurotic etiology: "In the middle of it, it [the self-analysis] suddenly ceased for three days, during which I had the feeling of being tied up inside (which patients complain of so much), and I was really disconsolate."[80] At this time, Freud thought of resistance as "arising from the masturbatory pleasure-seeking period of infancy that preceded the onset of repression," with the patient behaving like an obstinate malingerer until, Freud says, "I tell him so and thus make it possible for him to overcome this [infantile] character."[81]

Over time and with the elaboration of the structural theory, Freud came to understand better that resistance is part of the patient's illness and an intrinsic aspect of the defensive life of the ego. In his papers on technique, and later ones, Freud consistently stressed the importance of working with the resistance. For instance, in his last statement on the subject in *An Outline of Psycho-Analysis* (1940a), Freud wrote that "the overcoming of resistances is the part of our work that requires the most time and the greatest trouble."[82] However, as we pointed out in Chapter 1, Freud never used the term "analyzing" resistance, and he meant something else by working with resistance than does the contemporary clinician. In current psychoanalytic theory, analyzing resistance means exploring it fully for its own instinctual content, defenses, and conflicts. It is noteworthy that already in 1934 James Strachey, in his classic "The Nature of the Therapeutic Action of Psycho-Analysis," described the period in which Freud wrote his six technical papers (1911–1915) as the period of resistance *analysis*. This misapprehension is especially striking in view of the fact that Strachey, of course, was the main translator of Freud's work.

In Freud's theory and method, resistance was to be overcome, the German word for which is *überwinden*. Freud stated this idea early and clearly and never deviated from it. In the following section of "Remembering, Repeating and Working-Through" (1914a), which we referenced earlier, he elaborated his suggestions about the technique of handling resistance:

The first step in overcoming the resistances is made, as we know, by the analyst's uncovering the resistance, which is never recognized by the patient, and acquainting him with it. Now it seems that beginners in analytic practice are inclined to look on this introductory step as constituting the whole of their work. I have often been asked to advise upon cases in which the doctor complained that he had pointed out his resistance to the patient and that nevertheless no change had set in; indeed, the resistance had become all the stronger, and the whole situation was more obscure than ever. The treatment seemed to make no headway. This gloomy foreboding always proved mistaken. The treatment was as a rule progressing most satisfactorily. The analyst had merely forgotten that giving the resistance a name could not result in its immediate cessation. One must allow the patient time to become more conversant with this resistance with which he has now become acquainted, to *work through* it, to overcome it, by continuing, in defiance of it, the analytic work according to the fundamental rule of analysis.[83]

Freud writes of the *overcoming* of the resistance by the analyst's *uncovering* it. Strachey's translation here conforms exactly to the meaning of Freud's German,[84]—with the exception of the phrase "to become more conversant with this type of resistance," which literally translated from the original would read "to become engrossed in the resistance."[85] Working through the resistance does not mean, as it does today, that the analyst engaged in its lengthy exploration and interpretation but, rather, that the patient was to work *through* it by aggressively pushing through it, or acting in spite of it, and rededicating himself or herself to free association. The purpose of the analyst's interpretation of resistance is not to examine the content of the resistance or the nature of the anxiety underlying it but, rather, to point out to the patient that some behavior that he or she does not understand to be resistance *is* resistance. Armed with this fresh piece of knowledge, the analysand is strengthened in his or her ability to do work. The exhaustive exploration of the *how* and *why* of the resistance, which so preoccupies us in our work today, received far less attention. Freud's aim was to get the patient back to free-associating.

Freud's actual clinical behavior is consistent with his theory: in the case reports we also find that Freud did not, in the modern sense, *analyze* the resistance. As noted, he told Wortis, "I observed that you had a certain amount of *Widerstand* and I set about to remove it."[86] Resistance played an important role in all the treatments we have presented. Freud typically made his patients aware of the fact that they were resisting and often encouraged or even pressured them to give it up. Considering that the task of the treatment was to make the unconscious conscious, resistance *was* a hindrance; it stopped the patient from free-associating or otherwise complying with the requirements of the analysis. Freud conveyed this idea to Wortis when saying that soon Wortis's resistance would become clear so they could "attack it."[87]

A most important indicator of resistance was the disrupted flow of associations. Freud told Blanton that he was being superficial and that his self-reproaches were just a sign of resistance. On another occasion he told him: "You seem to be holding back something. . . . It is better not to prepare what you are to say.[88] When Freud noticed signs of resistance during H.D.'s analysis, he wondered whether she was once again preparing for her hours and thus compromising her ability to associate spontaneously. In Dorsey's case, the entire analysis seems to have focused on his resistance to free association; Freud called his tendency to intellectualize a "pseudoscientific orientation" and compared his associations to a "museum of psychopathology."[89] Freud wrote in his autobiography, "If the resistance is slight [the analyst] will be able from the patient's allusions to infer the unconscious material itself; or if the resistance is stronger he will be able to recognize its character from the associations, as they seem to become more remote from the topic in hand, and will explain it to the patient."[90] As we discussed earlier, free association signified task performance; resistance was equivalent to task avoidance.

There were other signs that indicated to Freud the presence of resistance—the patient's manner of speaking, for instance. Freud told Wortis: "You're always mumbling . . . it is sometimes used as *Widerstand*."[91] He said to H.D., "I can tell from the way you speak that you are hiding things. . . . You ran your articles together, you did not speak clearly."[92] Then there were the nonverbal cues. Blanton was told he was resisting because in addition to there being "something different in [his] voice," which Freud said prevented him from understanding him, Blanton covered his eyes and kept looking at his watch.[93] Resistance could also manifest itself in acting out against the boundaries of the treatment, such as being late. Wrote Wortis: "I was unfortunately late again. 'That means *Widerstand*,' said Freud." Wortis's remonstrations that he had good reasons were to no avail; Freud was "not altogether convinced."[94] H.D.'s acting out took the form of beginning late and ending early, behaviors that were interpreted by Freud as signs of resistance,[95] as were her worries over matters concerning the fee: "Freud thinks I have been worried in the unconscious," she wrote to Bryher, "about your paying my bills here, or about his asking more this time."[96] On the other hand, when the eager Blanton wanted to explain some somatic symptoms as resistance, Freud, after considering the possibility, suggested that it could just be the result of the heat.[97]

Freud often noticed resistance in dreams. For instance, although Blanton's transference seemed to be positive, Freud detected from a dream symbol that he was resistant to the treatment and told him, "Your dreams have been growing more and more obscure. This can only have one meaning: There is a change in the transference."[98] Wortis's resistance interfered persistently with the interpretation of his dreams.

Without conjecturing about its source, Freud frequently contented himself with simply pointing out the way resistance manifested itself. He told H.D. that he could see from signs that she did not want to be analyzed, that she was "hiding things,"[99] and that he "felt some sort of resistance."[100] She wrote to Bryher shortly after returning to Vienna: "Papa says I have set up a terrific resistance, it's some 'fear' he is anxious to get at."[101] And, without much success, Freud kept trying to convince Wortis that his intellectualizing was resistance.[102]

At other times, Freud combined pointing out to the patient the presence of resistance with an interpretation about its source. After noticing signs of resistance early in an analytic hour and making some initial suggestions that Blanton was perhaps bored or feeling that he was not getting his full hour, Freud finally concluded from a dream that Blanton harbored death wishes against him.[103] H.D.'s looking at her watch elicited several interpretations: "that I was not really happy on his couch, that I really wanted him to die, that I really wanted to die myself, that I really did not believe the analysis would help me and so on."[104]

At still other times, Freud tried to convince his patients through appeals to their will power and reason to give up their resistance. He said to Blanton in the beginning, "It takes time to develop the right attitude and to overcome resistance. But I am sure you will be of much assistance in helping us to overcome it."[105] This comment illustrates that, as we pointed out earlier, Freud had great faith in his patients' ability or willingness to adopt an attitude that would enable them to fight, or to speak in spite of, the resistance. This is reflected as well in Freud's criticisms of Wortis for not doing the work.

Freud often encouraged, or even pressured, his patients to overcome their resistances. He "scolded" H.D. for not being "eager enough to do psychoanalysis"[106] and told her that he was in charge of the clock: "I keep . . . time."[107] When Wortis's analysis seemed to be going nowhere, Freud threatened to end it right there. Wortis promised to cooperate more fully, but Freud was still irritated: "You ought to be ashamed of yourself for acting that way, grumbling and growling for three days because I said this or that to you. You will have to give up your sensitivity."[108] On other occasions he chided him for being late and for being too intellectual: "He then proceeded to criticize me roundly again for launching into abstractions."[109]

Freud expected his patients to be able to put their resistance aside and consider what he was telling them. When Wortis was unable to comply, Freud told him with annoyance that he was being unscientific: "An attitude of that sort makes further analysis impossible: it is purely emotional."[110] When Kardiner was defensive about Freud's interpretation concerning his relationship with his stepmother, Freud raised his voice and told him to give it up.

The work with resistance was an important aspect of every case reviewed here, as Freud had suggested it should be in his technical writings. Moreover, the clinical examples show that Freud considered resistance an interference with the task that the patient needed to give up through conscious effort so that the work (free association) could proceed.

ANALYSIS OF TRANSFERENCE

The analysis of the transference in Freud's procedure was used to support adherence to free association. It was not the primary method itself. Even though the following statement (which Freud addressed to Wortis) is about the positive transference, it seems to reflect Freud's view of the role of transference in general: "The psychoanalytic cure consists in bringing unconscious material to consciousness; to this end the positive transference is used, but only as a means to an end, not for its own sake."[111] Transference contributed to task performance by providing a potent motive for elucidating the nature of unconscious conflicts and by providing the basis for the therapeutic alliance that enabled the patient to face them. On the other hand, in its negative or erotic aspects it could become a major obstacle to treatment in the form of resistance. In his papers on technique, Freud stated unequivocally that analysis of the transference is an essential and central piece of the treatment. He wrote in 1914 that the compulsion to repeat is admitted into the transference as into a playground in which it "is expected to display to us everything in the way of pathogenic instincts that is hidden in the patient's mind."[112]

Freud differentiated the positive, or affectionate, transference from the erotic and negative. The importance of the positive transference lies in the fact that it attaches the patient emotionally to the analyst and thereby gives the analyst leverage for the work. As the foundation of the relationship and the force that motivates the patient to engage in the often difficult analytic work, it has a *synthetic* function and is therefore not analyzed. Freud wrote, "This *transference* . . . so long as it is affectionate and moderate, becomes the agent of the physician's influence and neither more nor less than the mainspring of the joint work of analysis."[113]

The clinical data show that Freud indeed did not analyze the positive transference and its derivatives except when he thought they served the purpose of resistance—hiding criticisms, competitiveness, anger, and the like. He questioned, for instance, the seemingly positive transference in Blanton's case after having noticed signs of resistance in his dreams. Dorsey commented as well, "Even my positive transference was resistance," without explaining, however, the particular meaning of this statement.[114] Freud interpreted Wortis's attempt to impress him as resistance and told him that his "professions of respect were just the familiar counterpart . . . to [his] real feelings."[115] On a later occasion Freud found that Wortis's apparent wish for conciliation seemed "*too* friendly and suggested an overcompensated hostility."[116]

Although Freud did not accept an apparently positive transference at face value, he missed its hidden meaning in some cases. Kardiner, for example, pointed out that his idealization of Freud covered up fear and anger, a mechanism he thought Freud missed in their relationship even though Freud had understood it precisely in Kardiner's analysis with Frink. In Kardiner's opinion, this was a major lapse on Freud's part. Perhaps it was an oversight, or perhaps Freud was not aware of any resistance in their relationship. It also appears that Freud interpreted the here-and-now transference less consistently, a point to which we will return.

There are instances in the case material that suggest that Freud tended to underestimate certain implications of his patients' attachment to and admiration of him—such as dependency needs and fear of loss— more than their hostile, competitive aspects. Comments such as those made by Freud to Blanton about his wish to be a family member and his wish for closeness are rare in these records.[117] Helene Deutsch illustrates this tendency with another example. One of Freud's favorite students, she had been in analysis with him for about a year (beginning in August 1918), when her analysis ended without warning. Freud told her unexpectedly and

> with absolute candor that he needed my hour for the "Wolf-Man," who, after an interruption, had come back to continue his analysis. Freud told me, "You do not need any more; you are not neurotic." . . . I considered myself mature enough then to react to the situation objectively, without bringing my transference problems to bear on it.[118]

Following this, Deutsch experienced the first serious depression of her life. It is interesting to note that Freud did not address his patients' transference reactions in any of the terminations: in fact, he seemed casual about many of the endings. Just prior to his termination of his analysis, Kardiner dreamed about a snowy Russian landscape, which Freud related to feelings about his mother's death. He did not make the connection to the fact that Kardiner was about to lose *him*.

Similarly, Freud did not seem to think that his failing health and frequent remarks about his death needed to be evaluated for their impact on his patients' feelings toward him. Money-Kyrle felt "appallingly depressed" following Freud's first cancer operations during his analysis: "But I did not see the connexion and I do not think he pointed it out."[119] Perhaps it was a blind spot; perhaps it shows again that Freud attributed less significance to the transference in the here-and-now than to projections from past relationships. But the fact that important possible transference implications were not consistently analyzed seems to confirm that transference did not play as central a role for the overall treatment as it does today.

Freud compared the secondary role of positive transference in psychoanalysis to the primary role of suggestibility in hypnosis. When transference is absent or entirely negative,

> there is also no possibility of influencing the patient by psychological means. It is perfectly true that psycho-analysis, like other psychotherapeutic methods, employs the instrument of suggestion (or transference). But the difference is this: that in analysis it is not allowed to play the decisive part in determining the therapeutic results. It is used instead to induce the patient to perform a piece of psychical work—the overcoming of his transference-resistances—which involves a permanent alteration in his mental economy.[120]

The comparison made here between the positive transference and suggestion explains further why Freud seemed to feel justified in trying to convince his patients to give up their resistances and accept certain truths. We pointed out earlier that he often challenged the strength and resiliency of an analysand's ego with the depth of his interpretations. Freud's conception of the positive transference may provide the missing link here: The attachment of patients to their analyst would enable them to rally their forces against the control and demands of the id and thus make use of their autonomous ego functions.

Freud has often been criticized for his use of suggestion in psychoanalytic treatment. De Saussure, whom we quoted earlier as saying that Freud was not a good technician, attributed Freud's use of suggestion to the fact that Freud had "practiced suggestion too long not to have been materially affected by it. When he was persuaded of the truth of something, he had considerable difficulty in waiting until this verity became clear to his patient. Freud wanted to convince him immediately. Because of that, he talked too much."[121] Freud did not disagree with the fact that he could be impatient, particularly toward the end of his career, when he wanted to spread the influence of psychoanalysis; nor did he disagree with the observation that suggestion, in the form of the positive transference, had a place in his treatment method. However, as he pointed out, suggestion in psychoanalysis, in contrast to its function in hypnosis, was not allowed to play a *decisive* role in accomplishing the task. In Freud's work the decisive role was played by free association.

While the positive transference was a prerequisite for successful treatment inasmuch as it engaged the patient in the work and gave the analyst leverage, transference in its other permutations could present a major obstacle in the form of resistance. Freud wrote that transference was the principal factor responsible for the breakdown of free association:

> When it has become passionate or has been converted into hostility, it becomes the principal tool of resistance. It may then happen that it will paralyse the patient's powers of associating and endanger the success of the treatment.[122]

In that case, it was analyzed and became a central focus. With Wortis, Freud noticed the negative transference primarily in his unwillingness to free-associate. But the transference resistance could manifest itself in other ways, for example, in Wortis's lateness or in H.D.'s checking the time frequently. Dreams often provided the clue. Blanton's increasingly obscure dreams indicated a change in the transference that Freud attributed to his having presented Blanton with the gift of his books. Wortis's wish that Freud's methods would fail did not escape Freud's attention and was interpreted from a dream.[123]

Freud handled the negative transference according to the same rules that applied to the handling of resistance and interpretations in general. He either simply pointed out its presence or added an explanation immediately. For instance, when H.D. entered his consulting room without looking at him in her first hour, Freud told her—even though it was "against the rules,"[124] that is, too early to be making interpretations— that she was disappointed in him. Freud's procedure here is in keeping with his theoretical prescriptions:

> The transference is made conscious to the patient by the analyst, and it is resolved by convincing him that in his transference-attitude he is *re-experiencing* emotional relations which had their origin in his earliest object-attachments during the repressed period of his childhood. In this way the transference is changed from the strongest weapon of the resistance into the best instrument of the analytic treatment.[125]

This statement points to another important difference between Freud's concept of transference and that of modern technique, namely, the relative weight attributed to transference as projections from the past ("re-experiencing emotional relations which had their origin in [the patient's] earliest object-attachments") versus transference as manifestations of the patient's current responses to the analyst, commonly referred to as the here-and-now transference. In contemporary theory and technique, the emphasis on the here-and-now transference coincides with a conceptualization of transference that comprises the totality of the analytic relationship. In contrast, Freud appeared to separate the relationship between analyst and patient into transference and real aspects; as Lipton (1977) pointed out, in Freud's technique it was only the transference relationship that was subjected to analysis. But even from his writings it is clear that Freud's purpose in analyzing patients' current reactions to their analysts was ultimately to demonstrate their infantile wishes and impulses toward original love objects.

Freud's theory is consistent with what we found in his treatments. The case material shows that he did interpret the current transference, although more in some cases than in others. There are numerous examples of his doing so in H.D.'s and Wortis's treatment. In the latter case, for instance, there was more emphasis on the current relationship because Wortis's resistance to free association and his obvious struggle with Freud made it immediately significant and perhaps because he revealed comparatively little about his past. Thus, Freud pointed out that Wortis was trying to steal from him and that Wortis disagreed with whatever he said and was being competitive with him.[126] Freud told H.D. in the beginning that she had come to Vienna—and to him—to find her mother. Money-Kyrle summed up his evaluation of Freud as an analyst with the following words: "Clinically, the most important difference was that Freud still set more store on the recovery of *memories* of traumatic experiences than on learning to understand the current complications of the unconscious and then working backwards to their source."[127]

Thus, after considering all the clinical data, it seems to us that the present relationship was not necessarily neglected or minimized by Freud; it is not a matter of choosing either past or present relationship but of recognizing their relative weights. However, it does appear that Freud's definition of and his work with the transference were narrower than is the case today, where the broadening of the definition of transference has shifted the focus increasingly into the here-and-now so that every aspect of the present relationship must be considered for its possible transference implications.

In the modern ideal, transference (along with resistance) analysis has become the engine of the treatment. In one prevalent version of this

ideal, analysts are required to be neutral so as not to disturb the transference projected onto their person; that is, they are relying upon the
analysis of transference rather than free association as their main method.
To put it differently, for the transference to be relived in the here-and-now
the analyst tries to allow a merging of the images of past and current
relationships by not becoming a real object to the patient.

This consideration was not significant for Freud because transference
analysis itself was not the primary means of accomplishing the task.
Moreover, he believed that being known to the patient as a real person
would not interfere with the development of the transference; indeed it
might facilitate it. Freud believed that the transference, as a projection
from the past and an important aspect of the patient's unconscious, would
necessarily emerge if the patient adhered to the prescription of free
association and that it would thus be repeated in the current relationship
regardless of the analyst's actual behavior; consequently, he believed he
could be himself *while* being a transference object. Recall the comment
he made to H.D.:

> "I do *not* like to be the mother in transference—it always surprises and
> shocks me a little. I feel so very masculine." I asked him if others had
> what he called this mother-transference on him. He said ironically and
> I thought a little wistfully, "O, *very* many."[128]

Freud, as well as his patient, could consider the projection onto him of
maternal transference as an inevitable part of the work, yet he could think
of it and treat it as separate from himself. He could, for example, be both
himself *and* the projected image of H.D.'s mother and could shift back
and forth between these two positions openly without regarding this
shifting as a hindrance. Cremerius (1981), commenting as well on the
division in Freud's clinical technique between real and transference
relationships, suggested that the inevitability Freud attributed to the
emergence of the transference onto the person of the analyst—regardless
of his or her behavior—explains why Freud thought it possible to analyze
his own daughter. Most recently, with the emphasis on concepts such as
projective identification, selfobjects, and intersubjectivity, the demarca-
tion between the real and transference relationships found in Freud's
technique is becoming further obscured.

MAINTENANCE OF NEUTRALITY
AND ABSTINENCE

Freud's analytic behavior has frequently been criticized for its lack of
neutrality and abstinence. The data in the present study clearly support

the observation that Freud was anything but a blank screen or mirror: He was visible and did not reflect back only what his patients showed him. In fact, his presence in the analysis was a strong one; he was real, authoritative, spontaneous, and personable. He talked to his patients about his passion for art, literature, and psychoanalysis. They knew how much he liked his dog and disliked nearly everything about the United States. He made no secret of the fact that he loved to gossip. His patients were often aware of his moods; he could seem bored, friendly, excited, angry, or impatient. Freud freely gave his opinions about books, people, and theories and did not hide his moral and political values. He introduced patients to his family; Bonaparte, for instance, was a good friend and visited the Freud family often in between her periods of analysis.

The question of whether or not he was neutral or abstinent was, within bounds, irrelevant for Freud. He was not concerned with particular behaviors or interventions for their own sake and did not care whether or not they were justified from a theoretical point of view. He was concerned with accomplishing the task. What mattered most of all was that the patient associated and the unconscious was being explored. As Lipton (1977) put it, Freud's behavior was secondary to its purpose. Interventions, within certain limits, were judged by their effectiveness, a view that is reflected in the statement he made in an early paper on treatment, written in 1905: "There are many ways and means of practising psychotherapy. All are good that lead to health."[129] Freud experimented. He said to Wortis, "You notice my methods with you have changed. I tried to use personal criticisms for a while, but you were too sensitive to it, and began to criticize me in turn, so that I have had to treat you more carefully."[130]

The question of countertransference must be considered here. As we have seen, Freud was often personally engaged with his patients. He clearly liked Kardiner but seemed to be indifferent toward Dorsey. He was often annoyed by Wortis and his stubborn refusal to take psychoanalysis seriously. He seemed fond of H.D. and treated her like the special daughter she wanted to be; in contrast to his adamant insistence with Kardiner that they terminate on the arranged date, he was flexible with H.D. about when to stop and more or less left the decision up to her. Since Freud was not trying to be neutral, there was no need for him to behave the same way with all his patients. Also, with transference analysis playing a more circumscribed role than is allotted to it today, Freud was freer than contemporary mainstream analysts to express countertransference. While he would have agreed that limiting the countertransference is a worthwhile goal, in practice he seemed to accept a good measure of it as an inevitable aspect of the analytic relationship. He chose to be real even if that meant revealing his own, at times exaggerated, feelings and reactions.

His patients, on the whole, did not seem to think that Freud's personal and real attitude interfered with the treatment. H.D. talked about an instance in which she and Freud strayed from their work by gossiping and talking about matters unrelated to the analysis; he quickly got them back to the task. Blanton was surprised about Freud's warmth and interest: "There was none of the cold detachment which I had imagined was the attitude an analyst is supposed to take. . . . Freud's manner made me feel secure and easy. At the same time, there was a detachment which was not repelling but pleasant." He added that this detachment "leaves you free to express yourself."[131] This was perhaps the most crucial point. In Blanton's opinion, Freud had "learnt the difficult art of countertransference. He gives of himself—but not indiscriminately or in a way that would burden the patient with the necessity of returning affection for affection, of like for like."[132]

The major concerns in Freud's technical suggestions that later hardened into the modern proscriptions regarding abstinence and neutrality were that patients not lose their motivation for change; that analysts put their own emotions aside if necessary to enable them to perform the task; that analysts not try to seduce their patients into giving up their resistances by revealing personal information; and that analysts keep their feelings under control in the case of an erotic transference. We will discuss Freud's theoretical guidelines with regard to these matters more fully in Chapter 8. In the cases presented here, there is no evidence that Freud acted in defiance of his own ideas.

Not being neutral, in some respects, was conducive to Freud's accomplishing the analytic task. It allowed him to be spontaneous, to make use of his associations, and to be actively engaged in his clinical work over several decades. For instance, taking H.D. to his study during an analytic session to inspect the various art objects helped "stabilize [her] evanescent ideas," an important consideration given her emotional lability;[133] with H.D.'s tendency toward being unreal and getting lost in her fantasy life, this kind of relating may have helped anchor her in the real world. Not being neutral further enabled Freud to be authoritative in the interest of the treatment and to clearly express values related to it, such as honesty and dedicated truth seeking.

Thus, it seems that for Freud the importance of working with the transference lay in the fact that it helped reconstruct the patient's childhood. The analysis of the transference therefore helped accomplish the task of making conscious the patient's unconscious infantile object relations. Freud believed that these ideas and fantasies from the past would necessarily emerge through free association even if he was real and not a blank screen. His personal engagement in the treatment could help advance the task because it allowed him to be active, directive, and authoritative. Most importantly, Freud did not believe that his lack of neutrality interfered with the treatment, the outcome of which remained his primary concern.

From Freud's Technical Suggestions to the New Orthodoxy

F ROM the beginning, psychoanalytic technique has been in a state of flux. Freud began one of his papers on technique, "Remembering, Repeating and Working-Through" (1914a), by describing in summary form the changes that had occurred from Breuer's cathartic method in the 1890s to the new division of labor in which the doctor devotes him- or herself to uncovering resistances to free association. Newer theories about the nature of mental illness and its treatment have amended, expanded, or, in some cases, altogether dispensed with Freud's technical suggestions. The transmigration of psychoanalytic practice from Europe to the United States following World War II further effected changes in the culture and institution of psychoanalysis that, we believe, had a major impact on psychoanalytic practice.[1] In this chapter, we examine the relationship between Freud's procedural advice and the current ideal of mainstream psychoanalytic technique in two aspects: one, Eissler's formulation of a model technique that has continued to exert powerful influence within the mainstream and among deviationist schools as well; and two, the conservative pressures of the American medical school as an organizational context for psychoanalysis. For a complete history of the evolution of psychoanalysis and its offspring psychotherapies in the United States, the reader is referred to Wallerstein (1995).

Our central point is this: In the three decades following Freud's death in 1939, American psychiatry became the primary locus for the institution of psychoanalysis with the consequence that Freud's technical guidelines were increasingly interpreted as rules derived from the objective scientific dimension of his suggestions. Notions of an ideal technique were postulated that were more absolute than Freud's had ever been. Most importantly, the analysis of transference and resistance came to replace free association as the technology of the treatment, and this technology (or method) was elevated to the status of a goal. The change both in the method and in the definition of the primary task had important consequences for the analytic relationship. Moreover, it was not understood that a change in task and technology was being advocated. Indeed, the modern version is often confused with Freud's technique, and the changes retrospectively attributed to Freud and called "classical."[2] Understanding how these changes took place and how the confusion about them occurred will add to our understanding of Freud and his technique in terms of both his theoretical formulations of it and his actual clinical practice.

In the 1977 paper referenced earlier, Lipton concluded that modern post-World War II psychoanalysis has expanded the concept of technique to include all aspects of the analytic relationship—in contrast to the approach practiced by Freud, who appeared to have distinguished between the transference and a personal, real relationship. It was only the transferential aspects, Lipton contended, that Freud subjected to analysis. The tendency of modern psychoanalysis to make procedure itself so all-encompassing had important consequences for the entire analytic situation. For example, it tended to shift the emphasis from the task of the treatment to the analyst's behavior so that his or her interventions were no longer evaluated in terms of treatment outcome but against abstract theoretical standards.[3]

Moreover, according to Lipton, modern technique prescribes that the analyst's responses be limited to interpretation of the transference neurosis. Concomitantly, silence and the absence of response have become defined as technically correct and usually exempt from the suspicion that the analyst is acting out, a suspicion that is applied to talking and other more active interventions. "When in doubt, keep quiet" is now a generally accepted prescription—yet a scrupulous analytic clinician is going to be in doubt most of the time. Lipton characterizes this procedure as "prophylactic" or "prospective" in that it is concerned with avoiding even minor interventions and the risk that they will become the subject of future associations. As a result, the analytic relationship has changed from "collaboration to unilaterality."[4] Both Lipton (1977) and Stone (1961) attribute the development of this modern technique to ego psychology and the controversy over Franz Alexander's procedural innovations at the Chicago Psychoanalytic Institute in the 1940s. We will discuss both points shortly.

The increasingly technical nature of the analytic relationship and the narrowing definition of what is procedurally correct behavior are importantly related to the new meaning assigned by Freud's followers to the concepts of abstinence and neutrality. But whether the issue is neutrality, the analyst's interventions, or the boundaries of the analytic relationship, one of the main points we want to stress here is the reductionism that has been employed in the interpretation of Freud's papers on technique. This trend had already become obvious during his lifetime, when Freud objected to the "docile," rule-bound analysts.[5] As modern techniques evolved, the ambiguity contained in Freud's suggestions on technique—flexibility versus rules—was collapsed in the direction of structure, objectivity, and formalism.

THE BASIC MODEL TECHNIQUE

Kurt Eissler's 1953 paper, "The Effect of the Structure of the Ego on Psychoanalytic Technique," has been so influential in the development of analytic technique in the United States that it has achieved the status of a classic. It demonstrates and is an important source of the changes we are describing in the structure of the analytic relationship. More general in tone than his earlier paper (Eissler, 1950) in which he criticized the technical innovations advocated by Alexander's "corrective emotional experience" (Alexander & French, 1946), the 1953 article presents Eissler's formulation of what he termed the "basic model technique." We prefer Eissler's term to Lipton's "modern technique" because although we are referring to an ideal we believe to be mainstream, we do not wish to suggest that it includes all modern thinking and practice.

Let us be clear at the outset that while we are critical of Eissler's basic model technique and especially of the chilling effect it has had on psychoanalytic thinking and practice over the years, there is much in his work that we agree with, especially his objection to analytic caprice and manipulation (whereby analysts act according to some theory of the patient's distant past that tells them what the patient "needs"). We, too, are for a disciplined approach. It should also be noted that Eissler himself pointed out that his basic model approach was an abstraction.

By way of introducing his 1953 paper, Eissler commented that he would discuss only one of the three variables that analytic technique depends on, namely, the patient's disorder and personality. He identified the other two critical variables as the patient's life and the analyst's personality, both of which he explicitly excluded, assuming for the sake of argument that they are "ideal" and that "no disturbance of the psychoanalytic process originates [from] either."[6] Eissler's willingness to exclude the analyst's personality from the discussion—even if it helps him argue his main points—is of great significance for the future definition of the analytic relationship, from which the person of the analyst increasingly disappears. It also allows for the creation of a completely abstract conception of treatment; that is, the treatment that is described is one that can never occur in reality. Eissler's model is so far removed from the grubby business of human relationships, including professional ones, that it functions more as a falsification than as a realistic ideal. Pure love, by contrast, is also an unattainable, if glorious, ideal, but real love does occur. No psychoanalysis takes place without the more or less disturbed (and changing, within the limits of analytic time) personality of the analyst. Nor does a psychoanalysis occur independent of the patient's life.

The role of the analyst in Eissler's model is similar to that of a scientist conducting an experiment in which he or she does not participate. In essence, this attitude can be seen as an extension or generalization of Freud's ideas regarding abstinence and analytic incognito and of his image of the analyst as surgeon. However, taken out of context and applied to the relationship and attitude as a whole, Freud's prescriptions lose their original meaning. Also, as we discussed earlier, Freud's surgeon metaphor stands in contrast to many of his other statements calling for flexibility and kindness—an attitude that did not find its way into Eissler's description of the ideal technique. Freud's suggestion that the analyst emulate a surgeon's detachment is meant to protect against the dangers of a *particular* technical difficulty; in Eissler's model it becomes the foundation, the point of departure, for the *entire* enterprise.

The scientific ethos of Eissler's 1953 paper finds expression not only in the emotional absence of the researcher but in its emphasis on rationality. Eissler's expressed intent for writing this paper was to "establish rationale and order into the psychoanalytic discussions of procedure and thus end the contemporary arguments, most of which [were] based exclusively on utilitarian viewpoints."[7] "Utilitarian" would here mean useful in accomplishing the task of the treatment, and we see in Eissler's remark the shift from Freud's emphasis upon the primacy of task to an emphasis on method. There may be people who would want a "true" psychoanalysis even if it could not help them, but had Freud thought analysis to be therapeutically ineffective in helping patients, he would have abandoned or radically revised it. The search for the cure of neurosis had inspired his professional and scientific exertions throughout the decade of his 30s and remained of great importance to him throughout the second half of his life even as his understanding of what constituted a successful analysis changed (Newton, 1995).

As the title of Eissler's paper indicates, the focus of his discussion and basic model technique was the ego and how the extent to which it is "modified"[8] or permanently damaged affects procedure. "A normal ego" is, Eissler writes, "one which, notwithstanding its symptoms, reacts to rational therapy with a dissolution of its symptoms."[9] Consequently, the extent of ego "modification" (or damage) and the true structure of the ego can be determined by its response to the model technique, not by symptoms or behaviors. In ideal psychoanalytic procedure, as Eissler sees it, interpretation is the only tool: "In the ideal case the analyst's activity is limited to interpretation; no other tool becomes necessary."[10] Occasional questions are the only exceptions. It appears that this is the origin of the notion that analysts should limit their interventions to interpretations of the transference neurosis. As Lipton (1977) writes, "[I]t may be that it was from this paper that a sort of myth arose, that is, that the analyst uttered no words except interpretations."[11]

EISSLER'S PARAMETERS

In the treatment of a patient whose ego is damaged, "parameters" may be introduced if strict guidelines about them are followed. A parameter is "a deviation, both quantitative and qualitative, from the basic model technique, that is to say, from a procedure which requires interpretation as the exclusive tool."[12] A parameter must be introduced only when the basic technique does not suffice, it must never transgress the unavoidable minimum, and its effects must be analyzable to the point where the basic model procedure can be resumed. The caution in the application of a parameter is due to the danger that "each parameter increases the possibility that the therapeutic process may be falsified."[13] The word "falsified" implies absolute notions of correctness and deviation, the latter being associated with departures from the model. Again, the sense is that what matters is not that the treatment succeed but that it be done correctly.

The introduction of the concept of parameter is very much in contrast to the notions of tact, flexibility, and experience, notions that were of such importance in Freud's suggestions and in his overall insistence that there are more ways than one to follow in questions of procedure. A parameter presupposes the existence of an ideal from which deviations regrettably occur; Freud never proposed the existence of an ideal approach. In Eissler's model, the analyst's involvement as a person is reduced and his or her activity limited to a small number of formalized interactions, thus narrowing the definition of what constitutes analytically acceptable or correct behavior.[14] In a panel discussion on "Variations in Classical Psycho-Analytical Technique," Eissler 1958 stated: "The science of interpretation is the bulk and main chapter of the classical psychoanalytic technique. Whether we interpret from the surface down or in the opposite direction, it is either correct or incorrect classical technique but not a variation of that technique."[15] Despite the fact that Freud refrained from confining matters of procedure to such a limited definition, Eissler claimed to base his notions concerning neutrality, abstinence, and analytically correct behavior on Freud's papers.

How representative or influential was Eissler and his basic model technique for modern psychoanalysis? The answer is that it was enormously important and came to represent *the* definition of classical psychoanalytic technique. As Wallerstein (1995) points out, the paper was "widely accepted as both the full establishment response to the threatening Alexander heresy and . . . the definitive version of the classical psychoanalytic technique inherited from Freud."[16] Reviewing the evolution of his thinking about technique during a conference in San Francisco in March 1996, the renowned American psychoanalyst Roy Schafer said that Eissler's parameters had put him in a "straight-jacket." And even though many analysts privately acknowledge that they practice differently from what the model prescribes, it is nonetheless remarkable that an ideal came into being that had these particular characteristics. Why should a model technique not include, as did Freud's, room for personal differences, flexibility, spontaneity, the analyst's personality, ongoing adult development, and such?[17]

EGO PSYCHOLOGY AND THE
AMERICAN MEDICAL ESTABLISHMENT

Let us return to the question of how this development in psychoanalytic thought can be explained. According to Stone (1961) and Lipton (1977), the increasing influence of ego psychology and the controversy over Alexander's technical deviations were determining factors in the development of the basic model technique. A third factor concerns the move of the organizational center of psychoanalysis to U.S. institutes—several of which were allied with prestigious medical school departments of psychiatry and teaching hospitals—and the development of a conservative branch that considered itself loyal to Freud but dependent upon the academic medical establishment.

Freud had trouble early on with the conservatism of these American psychoanalytic practitioners. In the 1920s he threatened to expel the New York Psychoanalytic Institute for its refusal to accept psychoanalysts who were not physicians. In keeping with his general view of things American, he viewed the New York psychoanalysts as second-rate and materialistic. When A. A. Brill, a leader of the New York Institute, learned of Freud's ire, he promised loyalty. Freud wrote Brill and told him that if the New York group should choose to defect, the international organization would lose nothing, scientifically or otherwise.[18] In "The Question of Lay Analysis" (1926a) Freud made is abundantly clear that he did not want "psycho-analysis to be swallowed up by medicine and to find its last resting-place in a text-book of psychiatry under the heading 'Methods of Treatment.' "[19] Since American medicine was not that eager to have psychoanalysis, some American psychoanalysts seeking a strong institutional base for psychoanalytic work tried to make it seem more like scientific medicine.

Lipton pointed out that the rise of the basic model technique seemed to coincide with the expansion of ego psychology. The title of Eissler's 1953 paper suggests the same conclusion, namely, that it was advances in the understanding of the ego that made clear which features of analytic technique were to be considered basic and which parameters. As noted, Eissler presented his basic model technique as classical rather than evolved.

We cannot provide a complete analysis of the role played by ego psychology in the rise of the basic model technique. Let us say briefly that the theory itself, even as expanded by Freud's followers, does not appear to provide a basis for major procedural revisions, especially the kinds of revisions described above. The primary implication of modern ego psychology for procedure relates to the handling of resistances; they are to be analyzed, not uncovered, overcome, and defeated. While Freud had introduced the idea of working with resistances long before the structural theory was formulated in 1923, he wrote consistently, as we have pointed out, of uncovering (*aufdecken*) and overcoming (*überwinden*), not analyzing (*analysieren*), them in the modern sense (see Gray, 1994). An emphasis on other factors also followed from an expanded ego psychology, including the patient's total personality, the nonconflictual sphere, adaptation to reality, and normal functioning (Hartmann, 1951). We should also note that ego psychology, like psychoanalysis generally, was not a theoretical monolith. Certainly Erik Erikson, the great psychoanalytic theorist of stages in ego development and of identity across the life cycle, was not Eisslerian in technique.

Freud never implied that his structural model required any changes in procedure (Lipton, 1977; Cremerius, 1981; Gill, 1982). Moreover, the further evolution of ego psychology after Freud still does not explain why it should have such a dramatic effect on the actual behavior of the analyst, as prescribed by Eissler. Gray (1994) pointed out that focusing on resistances requires more restraint on the part of the analyst in terms of giving up "a fascination with the id" and a "preoccupation with external reality including the past."[20] In some quarters, ego psychology not only has come to stand for the relinquishment of an active pursuit of id content, but represents a broader reaction against an id psychology that was associated with overinvolvement and narcissistic gratification on the part of the analyst, among other things. Moreover, in ego psychology there is perhaps an identification of the analyst's role with some of the ego functions whose development is being fostered, for example, secondary process thinking, rationality, structure, and defense against id impulses. Relevant as well here is Fenichel's (1938–1939) point of there being an oscillation throughout the history of analysis between an emphasis on analysts' intellect and rationality and an emphasis on their intuition and affect. Gray's (1994) emphasis upon cognitive learning as opposed to internalization in analysis, his eschewal of "interpersonal therapeutic ingredients," and his call for the creation of a "rational alliance" between analysand and analyst supported by the latter's "kindly scientific neutrality"[21] is the most recent influential expression of Eissler's emphasis on scientific rationality in treatment.

Even though modern ego psychology, with its emphasis on structure and rationality, does provide a different goal for treatment, it does not necessarily justify basic revisions in technique. It appears that both ego psychology and the increasingly formalized approach to procedure were affected by a general cultural preoccupation with scientific rationality and a specific preoccupation with scientific research and treatment within the American medical schools. A case in point is a statement by Eissler in which he explains his reason for creating high standards for technique, whether or not they can be adhered to in practice: "Whatever technique a therapist may devise can be used in the service of his pleasure principle. The value of a technical measure must rest on objective factors."[22]

FRANZ ALEXANDER AND THE
CORRECTIVE EMOTIONAL EXPERIENCE

Stone (1961) interpreted the emphasis on rationality in the basic model technique as a countertransference response to the overly personal therapies of Franz Alexander and others.

Alexander (Alexander & French, 1946) believed that the "corrective emotional experience" was the curative factor in treatment. He also argued that the therapist had to deliberately take roles and even decrease the frequency of sessions at times to force the patient out of a dependency upon the analyst and into a concern with the actual problems in living. He believed that neurosis resulted from a fault in interpersonal adaptation that had begun in childhood rather than, as Freud had argued, a fault within the personality that did not necessarily require environmental activation.

Alexander's technical proposals were troubling to many psychoanalysts because he considered the concept of the corrective emotional experience a legitimate evolution of Freud's ideas. Since he had been a disciple of Freud, he could claim sufficient legitimacy to stir up a discussion in the analytic community over the question of what constituted classical procedure. Analysts who thought of themselves as representing the classical point of view, such as Eissler, found Alexander's new formulations to be a deviation that threatened to undermine basic psychoanalytic principles. They criticized his technique as a regression to a prepsychoanalytic approach and the techniques of catharsis, suggestion, and trauma and as taking the place of what they had come to consider the primary tool, namely, analysis of the transference neurosis. According to Lipton, they claimed that Alexander "emphasized experience at the expense of insight, that he manipulated the transference rather than analysing it, and that he left unresolved a personal attachment which the patient developed to him."[23]

In response to what they considered an unacceptable deviation from psychoanalysis proper and to satisfy a need to define themselves in opposition to these kinds of new psychotherapies, analysts who called themselves classical asserted their position on a number of important technical and theoretical principles. In doing so, however, they were apparently unaware that they were redefining and reinterpreting Freud's statements and making them more rigid and orthodox in tone. Stone attributed the "extreme version of the concept of the analyst's noninvolvement in the patient's life, except in an interpretive sense," as it developed in the 1950s to "the pressures toward radical modifications of the psychoanalytic situation and techniques . . . , conspicuously those of Alexander and his coworkers, [that] have occasioned intellectual and scientific reactions in those convinced of the greater soundness and value of classical methods."[24]

This split in the psychoanalytic community was also reflective of some larger developments that occurred as a result of the center of psychoanalysis moving to the United States. Jacoby (1983) points out that there was a split between the mainstream, or orthodox, analysts and what he calls the revisionists, that is, theorists such as Erich Fromm, Karen Horney, and Harry Stack Sullivan. In his view, attempts to embed itself within the medical establishment (which continued to regard it with discomfort, suspicion, and even contempt) were costly to psychoanalysis in terms of its creative, revolutionary core. Haynal (1989) describes a breaking up into two camps: revisionists and those loyal to Freud. The loyalists ended up sounding more orthodox than Freud himself.

The reaction to Alexander in the 1940s and '50s was also part of a larger fragmentation within American psychoanalysis. Kanzer and Blum (1967) describe differences between the depth and structural schools as well as between older analysts who had come to psychoanalysis because of its revolutionary appeal and younger ones who saw it primarily as an interesting profession. The younger analysts tended also to be better grounded in the sciences than in the humanities, and so the humanistic aspect of psychoanalysis, so central to Freud's *Weltanschauung,* weakened. They lacked the classical education that had preceded Freud's scientific training in biology and neurophysiology and that was so essential to his discovery of psychoanalysis and to the manner in which he put these discoveries into practice. At the time of the Chicago school controversies, according to Kanzer and Blum (1967), psychoanalysis was entering an identity crisis. As noted, Fenichel wrote of the oscillation in psychoanalytic technique between overly intellectual and overly emotional approaches, and of the enduring argument among analysts about the dangers associated with either. In his view, psychoanalytic treatment in its early days tended to be too intellectual, whereas the kind of technique outlined by Ferenczi and Rank (1924) overcompensated for this tendency by proposing an excessively affective procedure. The Alexander–Eissler debate appears to be another instance of this conflict.

Even though the central roles of neutrality and abstinence—narrowly defined by Freud's followers in the manner described earlier—had already been called into question by the end of the 1950s, their influence on psychoanalytic procedure proved much more lasting. In a 1958 panel on psychoanalytic technique, a group of prominent psychoanalysts struggled with the question of what constituted standard technique and what constituted modifications or deviations from it. Eissler, on this occasion, reiterated his view that classical technique is one "in which interpretations alone have been used" but then, sounding less absolute—and more like Freud—concluded:

> We are better prepared to demonstrate errors and mistakes in an actual procedure than formulate a general code. Clinical multi-fariousness is much too great and the psycho-analytic theory of the personality still lags too far behind the clinical requirements of analytic practice to permit the establishment of laws that might serve as guides as reliable as the laws of physics or biology.[25]

Other analysts participating in this panel discussion defended interventions such as asking questions, answering questions, accepting gifts, or giving interpretations to resistant patients in the form of a joke. Nacht was among those challenging a rigid approach to neutrality and questions of technique in general. Considering the problem of therapeutic stale-mates, he wrote:

> I have noticed, however, not without astonishment, that we can be faced with the same difficulty [therapeutic stalemate] by taking the opposite course, that is to say by adopting rigidly, obstinately, and without question an attitude of absolute neutrality, and maintaining it strictly in despite of everything. . . . [C]ertain patients make endless use of these circumstances, which they feel as severely frustrating, in order to obtain a never-ending flow of masochistic satisfaction, no matter how good and accurate the 'interpretations' given them. I would add that these masochistic satisfactions sustain or feed certain unconscious sadistic tendencies which the analyst himself can experience. Thus within the analytical situation there is formed a sort of sadomasochistic 'couple,' an association which can become indissoluble if the patient develops a tenacious trans-ference neurosis.[26]

Nacht also pointed out that rituals rigidly adhered to may constitute a screen behind which the patient can hide certain aspects of his or her pathology. He suggested that analysts give up their neutrality when it threatens the treatment rather than furthers it and cease

> be[ing] the unchangeable mirror in order to adopt a new attitude of what I have called "presence." . . . I would point out here that it is not a question of the analyst using *some* new and carefully thought-out attitudes, but simply of emerging from the mythical world in which the patient likes to keep him, in order to enter into a life of reality and establish himself, *vis-à-vis* the patient, as adult to adult.[27]

Nacht had rediscovered an essential feature of psychoanalytic treatment, which Freud had always taken as a given and considered too obvious to mention—the real presence of the analyst as an adult actively involved with another adult in work.

THE RETURN OF THE RELATIONSHIP IN MAINSTREAM PSYCHOANALYSIS

In psychoanalysis the relationship, like the repressed, keeps coming back. One of Freud's earliest pivotal therapeutic discoveries, made in 1900, was that patients hung on to symptoms and resisted termination not because traumatic memories from childhood remained repressed, but because patients were attached to him by transference (see Newton, 1995).

Nacht's skepticism concerning analytic neutrality was echoed by an increasing number of analysts in the early '60s, with Stone being perhaps the most outspoken. In 1961, Stone described the troubling development in psychoanalytic technique that treated the " 'human' element" in the analytic relationship increasingly "as a sort of conscious détente, or reservation, or minimal forced concession."[28] He argued that this version was a misrepresentation of Freud's concepts of analytic incognito and abstinence, values that, Freud had cautioned, must not outdo the analyst's other concern, namely, "that neither the love nor the hostility reach extreme heights" in the transference.[29] In the basic model technique these concepts had become alienated from their original meaning, giving rise to superfluously remote and depriving attitudes that promote artifacts in the transference relationship:

> We must . . . concern ourselves with the absurd misinterpretations, exaggerations, or other misuses of the "mirror" concept indulged in by severely compulsive or self-indulgent personalities, or as a rationalization for passive cruelty, or through uncritical enthusiasm for what is thought to be the letter of the law.[30]

While detachment, unresponsiveness, and even coldness on the part of the analyst were sanctioned as correct behaviors by the modern definition of neutrality and abstinence, responses such as warmth, reassurance, and encouragement had become, according to Stone, *"bêtes noires"*; they were considered gratifying responses and were therefore to be avoided. With this observation, Stone made explicit an important point about the modern ideal, namely, that aggression in the analyst's behavior was more acceptable than love or nurture. Stone argued that to avoid every gratifying response can be as disastrous to the treatment as the attempt to substitute such responses for basic psychoanalytic tools. He, too, believed that the ambiguities and reservations found in Freud's statements had been interpreted in a one-sided fashion by proponents of the so-called classical position: "[R]ecent years have brought greater interest and attention to the 'human' side of the contradictory requirement," that is, detachment and involvement, sympathy and criticism.[31]

Stone pointed out that for Freud the justification for abstinence was to preserve the motivation for further change. Freud talked about abstinence for the first time in his 1915 paper on transference love. From the specific context of the erotic transference between a male analyst and a female analysand Freud generalized to the analytic situation as a whole:

> The treatment must be carried out in abstinence. By this I do not mean physical abstinence alone, nor yet the deprivation of everything the

patient desires, for perhaps no sick person could tolerate this. Instead, I shall state it as a fundamental principle that the patient's need and longing should be allowed to persist in her, in order that they may serve as forces impelling her to work and to make changes, and that we must beware of appeasing those forces by means of surrogates.[32]

In his 1919 paper "Lines of Advance in Psycho-Analytic Therapy," Freud continued with a more detailed discussion of the meaning of and need for abstinence in analytic treatment:

> By abstinence, however, is not to be understood doing without any and every satisfaction—that would of course not be practicable; nor do we mean what it popularly connotes, refraining from sexual intercourse; it means something else which has far more to do with the dynamics of falling ill and recovering.[33]

Abstinence, in Freud's theory, is an essential requirement of analytic work and refers to the withholding of gratification that is related to transference wishes and the effort to find relief from unconscious conflict: "The patient must be left with unfulfilled wishes in abundance. It is expedient to deny him precisely those satisfactions which he desires most intensely and expresses most importunately."[34]

In light of the letter from Freud to Ferenczi that we have quoted concerning the negative nature of his procedural advice, it is clear that Freud's warning here is directed against the danger of removing the motivation for change through an overly gratifying attitude in the transference: "Some concessions must be made to him, greater or less, according to the nature of the case and the patient's individuality. But it is not good to let them become too great."[35] What kinds of concessions can or should be made is left to the analyst's tact. In his 1961 book Stone remarks that the ambiguity regarding the exceptions gives little basis for inferring just what might be given to the patient, but he believes that Freud had in mind as necessary compensations such gratifications as sympathy and respect. With regard to the interpretation of this technical rule and of the ambiguities in particular Stone (1961) writes:

> [T]hose . . . , elements deriving naturally from the doctor–patient relationship, and persisting in the realm of common sense, . . . have been crowded increasingly to the theoretical and operational periphery—to be regarded as reservations, exceptions, or minimal necessary concessions, sometimes . . . taken for granted or optional or . . . downright errors.[36]

Two famous metaphors by Freud in his 1912 paper "Recommendations to Physicians Practising Psycho-Analysis"—in which the analyst is compared to a surgeon and to a mirror—have provided the theoretical justification for the neo-orthodox ideal. The surgeon analogy follows several other general suggestions about psychoanalytic treatment:

> I cannot advise my colleagues too urgently to model themselves during psychoanalytic treatment on the surgeon, who puts aside all his feelings, even his human sympathy, and concentrates his mental forces on the single aim of performing his operation as skillfully as possible. Under present-day conditions the feeling that is most dangerous to a psycho-analyst is the therapeutic ambition to achieve by this novel and much disputed method something that will produce a convincing effect on other people. . . . The justification for requiring this emotional coldness in the analyst is that it creates the most advantageous conditions for both parties: for the doctor a desirable protection for his own emotional life and for the patient the largest amount of help that we can give him to-day.[37]

Again, there is a context for Freud's statement that is much more specific than its usual interpretation suggests. Freud was concerned about the ill-effects of therapeutic ambitiousness. It was a temptation to which he himself had succumbed and against which he had subsequently learned to struggle in his early years as a young physician and private practitioner.[38] Therapeutic ambitiousness can interfere with the aim of treatment, as can other interests of the analyst, such as theory building, another matter Freud discusses in this paper just prior to using the surgeon metaphor. Freud's return to medical language and imagery may have been motivated by his concern that psychoanalytic treatment be distinguished from other psychotherapeutic methods. Stone (1961) interpreted Freud's statement to mean that a sympathetic attitude exists in the analyst but must be subordinated to the requirements of skillful technical work. With reference to the emotional coldness Freud advised, Stone understood this comment to be more a reflection of Freud's concern about the analyst's needs and frailties than a prescription of an overall attitude: "I see no reason . . . why this must in any sense be construed as a directive regarding a general personal attitude, in the larger sense. It would seem specifically applicable to the analyst's only scalpel, his interpretations, which may indeed, at times, be painful."[39]

The mirror simile appears in the same 1912 paper. Freud first discusses the temptation of an affective technique in which the analyst hopes to overcome the patient's resistance by talking about himself:

> Experience does not speak in favor of an affective technique of this kind. Nor is it hard to see that it involves a departure from psychoanalytic principles and verges upon treatment by suggestion. . . . The

resolution of the transference, too ... is made more difficult by an intimate attitude on the doctor's part, so that any gain there may be at the beginning is more than outweighed at the end. I have no hesitation, therefore, in condemning this kind of affective technique as incorrect. The doctor should be opaque to his patients and, like a mirror, should show them nothing but what is shown to him.[40]

According to Stone, here Freud is rejecting a procedural maneuver used to overcome resistances, a maneuver in which the analyst reveals the contents of his or her own mind in the hope that this will help elucidate the patient's thoughts. However, it is not an across-the-board principle: "There is no evidence that 'coldness' or 'lifelessness' were directly or indirectly adjured in this particular recommendation; it is purely of cognitive-communicative reference."[41] If this recommendation were accepted literally, Stone argued, it would be incompatible with the essential nature of psychoanalysis, since interpretations are necessarily subjective; moreover, it is incompatible with other comments Freud made about the necessity of friendliness and sympathy on the part of the analyst.

THE NEUTRALITY APOCRYPHA

In the evolution of the concept of neutrality, so important to the basic model technique and as an ongoing ideal, there has been a tendency to interpret out of context the meaning of particular suggestions by Freud concerning the analyst's attitude and to generalize from them. The concept of neutrality, as well as the term itself, is thought to have originated in Freud's 1915 paper "Observations on Transference-Love," the last of his "recommendations to physicians" series. Remarkably, reading Freud's paper in German reveals that he did not use the word "neutrality." In the context of discussing how erotic transferences should be handled in the treatment, Freud states that the analyst should not "deny" the "indifference" he has acquired by "keeping his countertransference in check" (our translation).[42] Strachey translated the word *Indifferenz* as "neutrality," even though there is a German word, *Neutralität*—which Freud did *not* use—that translates directly into its English cognate.[43]

The fact that Freud chose *Indifferenz*, a loan-word of Latin origin that is much less commonly used in German than *Gleichgültigkeit*, meaning "indifference" or "disinterest," is noteworthy. *Gleichgültig* suggests an attitude more uncaring than we believe Freud was recommending. Furthermore, the use of Latin, which Freud generally avoided, may have been meant to suggest, as did the earlier surgeon analogy, the desired professional demeanor in the face of a temptation like erotic transference. The word *Indifferenz* suggests an acquired—in fact, Freud uses the word *erworben,* or, in English, "acquired"—mental position and implies an underlying emotional participation on the part of the analyst that involves vulnerability to such matters as falling in love with patients. The term "neutrality," from the Latin *ne-uter* ("neither") is, in contrast, spare of meaning; it is a generic, colorless word. The combination of the particular context in which Freud's remark is found and the linguistic nuances makes this paragraph of Freud's recommendations an intriguing example of his deeply sympathetic attitude toward both patient and analyst and their human weaknesses, which have to be controlled in the interest of the treatment.

This sympathy or emotional resonance is manifested a few pages later in a startling and little-noted phrase in which Freud writes that it is perhaps the subtler romantic implorings that are most likely to lead the analyst to abandon the task in favor of "a fine experience."[44] Actually, Freud was imagining *"ein schönes Erlebnis"*—*"a beautiful experience."*[45] There being no linguistic justification for translating *schönes* as anything other than "beautiful," one sees again the yearning for asepsis, this time on Strachey's part. Fine experiences are very nice indeed, but a beautiful one can change one's life for good (or bad). Beautiful, deadly experiences lurk in the worlds imagined by Thomas Mann in *Death in Venice* and *Doctor Faustus* or by Vladimir Nabokov in *Laughter in the Dark* or *Lolita.* A fine experience is what Tiny Tim had with the roast goose in Dickens's novel *A Christmas Carol.* The word "neutrality" is devoid of these dark implications of emotional danger and bears little resemblance to the original meaning of Freud's statement.

The later interpretation of Freud's concepts of abstinence and neutrality was a far cry from his original prescriptions, let alone, as we have seen, his actual clinical behavior. To quote Stone (1961):

> The early development of the psychoanalytic situation moved toward an extreme version of the concept of the analyst's noninvolvement in the patient's life, except in an interpretive sense. This excluded even professional reactions to or interest in symptomatic suffering as such, or concern with the duration of treatment, or other matters which are usually within the routine scope of medical consideration, and, of course, always of profound interest to the healthy portion of any patient's personality. 'Only to analyze' or an equivalent phrase became a sort of catchword or slogan for the definition and circumscription of the analyst's function, and often, by implication, of his personal attitude.[46]

Ralph Greenson, a mainstream psychoanalyst who devoted himself in his writings to getting the real relationship back into psychoanalysis described a chilling example of what Stone was writing about. A young analyst Greenson was supervising presented an analytic hour of a woman whose baby was ill. She told her analyst how frightened she had been during the night when her son was running a high fever and having convulsions and she was unable to reach her pediatrician. The young analyst made no response of any kind, and when his patient fell silent, he told her she was resisting. He later told Greenson that he thought her silence represented a resistance to her own death wishes toward her son and that he was waiting for the revelation of such wishes to come up on its own. When Greenson told the analyst that the woman's realistic distress required some kind of response from him, he "primly reminded [Greenson] that Freud had said we are not supposed to gratify our patient's instinctual and narcissistic wishes."[47] During the next hour the woman wept silently and the only words exchanged were an occasional inquiry from the analyst as to what she was thinking. Greenson asked the analyst if he had found out what happened to the baby. He had not. Greenson told his supervisee that the analysis could not succeed in the emotional climate created by his own inhumanity; indeed, during the next meeting the patient quit.

In the 1960s, criticism such as Stone's and Greenson's was increasingly directed against the rigid, overly rational, detached attitude thought to be classical. Some of Freud's ideas that had been lost in the reformulation of technical principles found their way back into the repertoire of acceptable procedure indirectly through what were taken to be new concepts in new theories. Examples are the central place given to empathy in self psychology; the popularity of notions such as Winnicott's "holding environment" and Greenson's "real relationship" and "therapeutic alliance"; and the widened use of parameters, which found theoretical justification in object relations theory and made possible the psychoanalytic treatment of deeply disturbed patients. The expressive freedom in the role of psychoanalyst as exemplified by Lacan's dramatic escape from the straitjacket of the basic model technique is another example of strenuous modern efforts to expand the analyst's role to the dimensions Freud originally gave it. Finally, there is the contemporary excitement for and against the idea of intersubjectivity.

This is not to say that these theories have nothing new to offer but, rather, that they attempt unwittingly to restore the original unity of Freud's procedure. It shows just how little is actually known about Freud's technique when empathy on the part of the analyst as an important therapeutic factor is treated as if it were a new discovery or when intersubjectivity is represented as a deviation. What softer empathy shall we find and what subjective union more intimate than Freud's instruction that the analyst "bend his unconscious like a receiving organ around the transmitting unconscious of the patient"? Can we get closer without facing ethics charges?

In summary, a major departure from Freud in the basic model technique is its conceptualization of the analytic attitude, especially in terms of abstinence and neutrality. The stance of analyst toward patient in this model technique is much more formal and the analyst's behavior is more strictly regulated according to exact standards than Freud ever suggested. These standards are in keeping with the scientific-rationalist approach Freud adopted at times with respect to procedural matters. But, unlike Freud, those who subscribe to this modern position elevate this approach to an all-encompassing principle while the other end of the pole—the subjective, intuitive, spontaneous dimension—is lost. This imbalance affects not only the analytic attitude per se, but the entire relationship. It also affects the growth of knowledge about technique. The personal participation of the analyst cannot really be removed from the treatment situation, and the attempt to do so theoretically can only mean that it must continuously reappear in the form of "new" schools and theories.

THE EVALUATION OF FREUD'S CLINICAL TECHNIQUE BY MODERN STANDARDS

Some of the changes in psychoanalytic procedure described in the preceding pages have distorted not only our knowledge of Freud's theory of technique but also our understanding of his actual clinical behavior. This confusing development can be traced to three factors. First of all, as noted, the new standards that had been established for the basic model technique in the 1950s were erroneously attributed to Freud. This was possible because they were, in part, based on Freud's original suggestions and therefore could be represented as an extension of his ideas. Moreover, the authors of the new procedure considered themselves classical analysts and believed that they were merely contributing to the purification of Freud's psychoanalytic method, which was becoming diluted and adulterated by revisionists. Lipton (1977) commented on this lack of distinction between Freud's and the neoclassical techniques:

> [T]his [Freud's] technique was accepted as classical for some 40 years, and subsequently it was repudiated and replaced by a different tech-

nique also called, confusingly, 'classical' and still more confusingly, identified with a presumed later development in Freud's own technique which in fact never occurred.[48]

Second, the erroneous attribution of the modern ideal of procedure to Freud made it now seem as though a discrepancy existed between his theory and his clinical behavior. His treatment behavior was, quite obviously, not in accordance with the new standards of technique. Until this time, Freud's clinical behavior had been accepted as standard; now it was dismissed as being deviant from his own prescriptions.

Third, the apparent contradiction between his theory of technique and his behavior in practice was resolved in favor of the theory, which was considered to represent more accurately Freud's real position on the subject. Concomitantly, his actual clinical procedure was either ignored altogether or devalued; it was regarded as obsolete, even an embarrassment, and was not studied in its own right. In comparison to the basic model technique, Freud's method was called unanalytic, capricious, and haphazard. The criticism that Freud was unorthodox highlights the confusion regarding who should have the authority to decide what is true psychoanalytic technique. The word "orthodox" (from the Greek, meaning of "right or true opinion") in this context lends itself to the confusion. The right or true opinion could refer either to what is traditional or to what is currently accepted. Yet it seems absurd and arrogant to say that Freud was unorthodox or that he was not psychoanalytic. If we wish to do things differently from the founder, we ought to have the courage to name these innovations after ourselves. The belief that Freud's method was outdated had become so prevalent that many authors contented themselves with showing just that.

THE RAT MAN

Judging Freud's technique from the point of view of later standards has led several authors to conclude that his technique is now outdated or preclassical, implying that it has no relevance for contemporary thinking. Freud's treatment of the Rat Man, which occurred in 1907 (when Freud was 51), is often the basis of these latter-day critiques in part because we have the notes that Freud wrote about the case as it was actually under way. This is the first real glimpse we get of his clinical work after the Dora case, which he conducted in 1900. In the Dora case Freud had in hand the various elements of his mature therapeutic technique, although, as he said when he published it in 1905, he was still struggling to master the handling of the transference. His first papers on technique would not be written for another several years. In the following pages we briefly describe the case of the Rat Man.

The Rat Man was a college-educated man of about 30 whom Freud began treating for tormenting obsessions, irrational fears—including the astounding worry that his father, whom he knew to be dead, would die—and compulsive behaviors. The treatment lasted about a year and was successful in removing the symptoms and restoring the patient to a state of health. Freud dubbed his patient the Rat Man because these rodents figured in his central obsessive fantasy, namely, that rats might bore into his anus or those of his loved ones.

The Rat Man quickly developed a strong transference to Freud, one with marked ego-alien anal aggressive content, and analyst and patient were soon highly engaged in their work together. The flavor of the engagement can be evoked from a quote from Freud's account of their second analytic hour. The first sentence of that account shows once again the tremendous importance Freud placed on free association: "The next day I made him pledge himself to submit to the one and only condition of the treatment—namely, to say everything that came into his head, even if it was *unpleasant* to him, or seemed *unimportant* or *irrelevant* or *senseless*. I then gave him leave to start his communications with any subject he pleased."[49] Not much later, the patient began an hour by offering to tell Freud the event that had occasioned his coming for treatment. His obsessions had troubled him since childhood, but two months earlier, while on maneuvers with the army, he met a Czech officer who struck him as sadistic. This officer began to tell the patient of a peculiar form of punishment used in the East. Freud wrote:

> Here the patient broke off, got up from the sofa, and begged me to spare him the recital of the details. I assured him that I myself had no taste whatever for cruelty, and certainly had no desire to torment him, but that naturally I could not grant him something which was beyond my power. . . . The *overcoming* of resistances was a law of the treatment, and on no consideration could it be dispensed with.[50] (italics added)

Nonetheless, Freud offered to help give voice to the unspeakable by guessing the words his patient found too awful to utter. "Was he perhaps thinking of impalement?" Freud asked.

> "No, not that," the patient answered, "the criminal was tied up . . . a pot was turned upside down on his buttocks . . . some *rats* were put into it . . . and they"—he had again got up, and was showing every sign of horror and resistance—" . . . *bored their way in* . . . "—Into his anus, I helped him out.[51]

Freud was very aware of the Rat Man's transferences, at least in the first four months covered by his raw case notes. Freud called these "treatment-transferences" and watched them closely. However, the patient's actual life—present, adult past, and childhood—received close attention along with the transferences. These notes show Freud explicitly asking himself questions, posing hypotheses, rejecting some and accepting others. He did this not merely in private but also collaboratively with the patient. At times Freud was openly appreciative, even admiring, of the patient's good psychological ideas. Thus, as we saw with H.D. and the other patients, he made the Rat Man a reasoning collaborator in the work, not just a producer of material or data.

When we read these notes with an evenly hovering attention, we came to a surprising discovery: In a seeming paradox, Freud was both more authoritative and more collaborative than many modern analysts, who nonetheless imagine that by eschewing the overt exercise of authority (by, for example, avoiding making the fundamental rule explicit) they are being kinder, more empathic, or egalitarian. Gray (1994), for example, is at pains to rid the analyst of authority, making no distinction between being authoritative and being authoritarian. In criticizing Freud's approach to resistance, he goes so far as to describe it as relying upon the "authoritative, hypnotic-suggestive influencing potential of transference in overcoming resistance."[52] Gray wants the relationship between analyst and patient to be a collaborative one, and like many other contemporary analysts but unlike Freud, Gray views authority and collaboration as incompatible. Unfortunately, the analyst's authority is given in social reality and cannot be defined out of existence (see Newton, 1971, 1973a, 1973b, 1989, 1992a).

The sense one gets in reading this case and others is that analyst and analysand are working on a joint project or that their two separate tasks are united in the treatment—the Rat Man's task being to dispel with understanding the tormenting irrationality of his obsessions and Freud's being to understand the nature of obsessive–compulsive neurosis. Here again we see that when Freud analyzed a patient he was engaged simultaneously in a clinical and a research endeavor, though with an awareness of their points of departure, as when in "Recommendations to Physicians Practising Psycho-Analysis" he warns against the formal scientific study of a case while it is under way.[53] Recall Freud's excitement with H.D. over the new insights he was gaining about the role of the mother in the development of girls. For the great majority of clinicians, treatment is not concurrent with scientific study; clinicians are trying simply to help their patients, earn a living, and get better at their craft. Since they are not actively engaged in the larger project of advancing knowledge, a source of vital engagement, so important to Freud, is missing from their practice.

Freud engaged in other deviations from the basic model technique in addition to filling in some of the blanks in his patients' utterances. He requested that the Rat Man bring in a picture of his girlfriend, whose name the patient had refused to divulge, a request that produced a brief storm of resistance followed by acquiescence. On another occasion the patient had a perverse, ego-alien transference fantasy that he refused to describe. In an attempt to overcome the resistance, Freud explained the theory of transference to him and lectured a bit on perversions. During the third month of the analysis, the Rat Man broke off his free associations by deciding to give Freud a historical account of his obsessions. Freud welcomed this; from time to time he was glad to leave the business of free association and talk in other ways.

Perhaps Freud's most famous parameter in the Rat Man case was giving him a meal. His notes read simply, "He was hungry and was fed." Freud had had a meal prepared for his patient, which was evidently consumed in the consulting room during the patient's normal treatment hour. Not surprisingly, this act produced a transference reaction, which Freud was happy to analyze, revealing the remarkably paranoid fantasy that the purpose of this prandial interruption was to prolong the analysis. Not content with feeding his patient, Freud also offered him an observation on female grooming. When the patient spoke of seeing his girlfriend's pubic hair while she was lying on a sofa, Freud lamented that women no longer devoted attention to the grooming of their pubic hair since they now considered this growth to be unsightly.

Zetzel (1966) viewed Freud's serving the Rat Man a meal as "unanalytic," an act that, she noted simultaneously, did not impede "the progress of this patient's treatment."[54] Despite praising Freud's work with the Rat Man and stressing the priority of therapeutic alliance over therapeutic procedure, Zetzel nonetheless needed to opine that Freud's technique "differed considerably from his later theoretical models—his communications were not limited to interpretation of the transference neurosis."[55] She continued, "A good analytic situation, although it may temporarily be distorted or modified, will not be undermined by occasional defects from *traditional technique** on the part of the analyst [italics added]." The asterisk was added by the editors, Bergmann and Hartman, who included Zetzel's paper in their book on psychoanalytic technique, and refers to their footnote directing the reader to the 1953 paper by Eissler for a "more rigorous approach to the problem of deviation from the standard technique."[56] The editors also chide Zetzel for being deferential toward Freud's technique and weigh in themselves to criticize Freud's treatment of the Rat Man as outmoded and merely psychotherapeutic, a corrective emotional experience rather than true psychoanalysis, in its failure—among others—to analyze the patient's relationship to his mother.

The idea that analysts should limit their responses to interpretation of the transference is, as noted, a tenet of the basic model technique.

Much of modern analytic treatment in fact proceeds not as Freud's cases did—by free association and counterassociation—but by analysis of the transference and resistance; indeed, *Analysis of Transference* is the title of a highly regarded and widely read work by Merton Gill (1982). Yet Freud never said anything of the kind. Moreover, in addition to making assumptions about Freud's theory on technique, Zetzel neglected to reconcile her observation that despite Freud's extraneous responses and interventions a positive therapeutic alliance was established with the Rat Man.

Robert Langs, also a critic, at least understood that Freud deviated not from his own standards but from ours, even as he, too, uses the term "classical" confusingly. Langs (1980) wrote of the "misalliance between Freud and his patients, and its relationship to deviations in technique as measured by the template of current psychoanalytic standards."[57] His findings about Freud's procedure in the Rat Man case are as follows:

> There are two types of deviations from current classical technique. The first concerns the nature of the interventions that Freud made and, in general, reflects deviations in Freud's neutrality, level of activity, and degree of anonymity. The second includes specific deviations in technique such as feeding the Rat Man and lending him a book.[58]

In his analysis of the Rat Man case, Langs cites numerous deviations, or what he calls "frame violations," in Freud's treatment of the Rat Man as well as in his other case studies.[59] Most remarkably, in his analysis of the data Langs, like Zetzel, fails to take into account the fact that the treatment of the Rat Man was successful despite the alleged violations. This is not to say that the positive treatment outcome should obviate a thoughtful examination of the process by which it was achieved. However, it at least raises the possibility that perhaps other factors in Freud's technique were more significant than adherence to a post-Freudian conception of therapeutic structure. Langs's explication, which focuses narrowly on perceived procedural violations, misses the point that the patient improved; thus, he sheds little light on what Freud did to achieve success. Note again the displacement of the task of treatment by an emphasis on method: What matters most is not helping the patient but behaving correctly.

THE WOLF MAN

Freud's procedure as evidenced in his case histories is often criticized for failing to deal adequately with the transference and countertransference

(Kanzer, 1952, 1980; Glenn, 1980). Weiss (1980), for instance, criticized Freud's technique in the Rat Man case and called it preclassical because of Freud's limited understanding of transference, countertransference, ego defenses, and the superego. Rangell (1974) went so far as to assert that the analyses of the Rat Man and Wolf Man are now obsolete and we concede that they certainly are over. Holland (1969), trying to justify Freud's unconventional way of treating H.D., was not sure it even deserved to be called psychoanalysis: "The analysis (or whatever you wish to call it). . . ."[60]

The case of the Wolf Man has frequently been used as a foil for revisionist critique. Here again, Freud offers only glimpses of his work. He intended the piece not as an explication of therapeutic technique or even of adult psychopathology but, rather, of the manner in which an adult's disabilities can be built upon a preexisting infantile neurosis—thus the title of the paper, "From the History of an Infantile Neurosis." Freud called his patient the Wolf Man because of a nightmare the patient had had as a child of being watched by wolves sitting in a tree. Freud and the patient would discover that the silent, rapt attention of the staring wolves stood for the patient's own attitude when as a small child he witnessed the primal scene.

Roughly 25 years of age, the Wolf Man first presented to Freud in 1910 with a long history of serious mental illness.[61] His chief complaint was that the world was hidden from him in a veil, or that he was separated from the world by a veil, a condition that sounds like dissociation. Only one thing, which occurred but infrequently, removed the veil and restored the immediate experience of being alive—a bowel movement. The patient had been notably phobic and obsessional as a child; following a gonorrheal infection at 18, he had become incapacitated. By the time of his treatment with Freud, he had been in and out of sanatoriums with a diagnosis of manic-depressive psychosis and was largely unable to care for himself.

The first phase of the treatment lasted four years, until 1914. For a long while the patient was superficially compliant but subtly resistant. He was entrenched behind an attitude of what Freud called "obliging apathy."[62] For months, perhaps years, little change occurred. "It required," Freud wrote, "a long education to induce him to take an independent share in the work"; once he did, the relief that resulted became a new point of comfortable fixation.[63] Finally, as a way of forcing the resistance to the surface, Freud made an intervention for which he has been harshly rebuked. He told the patient that his chronically constipated bowel, which ordinarily could not function without enemas, would soon begin to move on its own. The Wolf Man greeted this prediction with the frank incredulity that Freud had hoped to expose. "I then," Freud wrote, "had the satisfaction of seeing his doubt dwindle away, as in the course of the work his bowel began, like a hysterically affected organ, to 'join in the conversation,' and in a few weeks' time recovered its normal functions after their long impairment."[64]

Now this would seem at bottom, if not on the face of it, to be a contribution to the patient's well-being of sizable proportions. Yet since it was achieved by suggestion, Gedo and Goldberg (1973) complained that "this intervention was never resolved through interpretation, [and therefore] the technique of the treatment cannot be viewed as psycho-analytic from today's vantage point."[65] Again we note the subordination of task performance to methodological correctness in modern evaluations.

In a further effort to overcome what we would now call the patient's character resistance, Freud introduced a yet more shocking parameter in his treatment of the Wolf Man. In an effort to help overcome the Wolf Man's resistances, after three years of treatment, Freud set an arbitrary termination date a year hence. He made clear that the date would be kept regardless of the progress achieved. The patient came to see that Freud was in earnest, and "under the inexorable pressure of this fixed limit his resistance and his fixation to the illness gave way, and now in a dispro-portionately short time the analysis produced all the material which made it possible to clear up his inhibitions and remove his symptoms."[66] Note again that the resistances were *overcome*, not analyzed in the modern sense. The treatment was terminated, but later, following World War I, Freud saw him again and found that there remained transference residuals that required further analysis. In 1926 the Wolf Man resumed analysis briefly with Ruth Mack Brunswick, who determined that he was in relatively good health despite some neurotic sexual problems and despite the fact that the war had left him impoverished. She maintained contact with the Wolf Man afterward, and he continued to tolerate the vicissi-tudes of life, some of which were dramatic, without relapse into serious psychopathology.

CONCLUSION

Authors tend to view the work with the Wolf Man and others as effective only because of Freud's brilliance and the power of his personality, not to the merits of the procedure itself. Such a view is common and is reflected in this statement by Weiss (1980) about Freud's treatment of the Rat Man:

> Such shortcomings (in dealing with the transference, countertransfer-ence, superego, etc.), which would soon be overcome, do not detract

from the genius, intuition, and creative ability that Freud showed in mastering practical as well as theoretical problems presented by this case of obsessional neurosis.[67]

Conclusions like these are an attempt to explain why Freud's "mistakes" frequently do not appear to have interfered with the success of the treatment and are, in effect, condescending. And the message for the rest of us mere mortals is clear: Stick to the rules.

CHAPTER NINE

Conclusions

I F current practices are a reaction to what has gone on before—and this must be the case in science and scholarship since these are public, partially cumulative endeavors—then to the extent that we misunderstand the past must we be confused about what we are doing now. We have tried to show that the reigning assumptions about orthodoxy and deviance in psychoanalysis arise from misunderstandings about Freud's work. Although not the focus of this book, there are also unresolved arguments about the essential differences between psychoanalysis and psychoanalytic psychotherapy. For us, what makes a treatment psychoanalytic is neither the frequency of meetings nor the manner in which the participants are seated but, rather, the division of labor that exists between them. We have found that the division of labor in Freud's treatment differed importantly from the mainstream ideal that has affected much of modern practice and that these differences have been poorly understood. We do not insist that Freud's way was correct and evolved approaches are erroneous but, rather, that getting clearer about the differences helps us become more conscious of the choices we are making in going about our clinical work. If one wishes to try Freud's way, the realm of choice about how one may relate to patients expands. Ultimately, within legal and moral limits, that division of labor is best that most effectively accomplishes the task. Yet the definition of the primary task of a psychoanalytic treatment can, sometimes imperceptibly, vary in consequential ways from one theorist to another, from one treatment to another, and between doctor and patient. Moreover, task accomplishment in any enterprise devoted to the psychological development of a person is intrinsically difficult to assess. Values, politics, careerism, and genuine methodological conundra ineluctably cloud efforts at assessment, essential as such efforts are.

FREUD'S DIVISION OF LABOR

The basic elements of the division of labor in Freud's psychoanalysis are that the patient free-associates and the analyst counterassociates, usually silently; when audible, the analyst's utterances range from raw counterassociations to organized interpretations in which the counterassociations are combined with other material. By *basic* elements in the division of labor, we mean, as Freud did, that this is the underlying structure of the interaction, the one to which a return from excursion is always made, not that free association and counterassociation happen every minute. This division of labor necessarily produces a deepening and widening of experience for both analyst and patient. Patients learn more about themselves and their lives—childhood and adult pasts, the present, and imagined futures. Analysts learn about these aspects of their patients and about people generally, including themselves, and they learn more about psychoanalysis. Perhaps of equal importance, patients take from their treatment a powerful tool for staying in touch with themselves and for maintaining a dynamic integration in the future—free association, which can be done silently or out loud selectively with intimates.

In Freud's approach, analysts are free to express themselves more fully because they are not relying on incognito and mirror effects to generate and protect an analyzable transference but, rather, are depending upon free association. The transference occurs as a result of an explicit division of labor and is not dependent upon the analyst's creating an aura of mystery or otherworldliness by behaving in ways that are socially strange. Thus, the transference may seem more real to the patient; it is harder to dismiss as an artifact or product of the peculiarities of the analyst's behavior. Freud found, as we have also in our own work, that the transference is quite sturdy. If the analyst's behavior has produced a transference reaction, this can be usefully analyzed; patients still respond to the reality of their analyst's behavior in their own distinctive ways, as the Rat Man did when he concluded that Freud had served him a meal as a means of wasting some of an analytic session and thus prolonging his treatment.

Freud's division of labor is essentially different from the division of labor in the basic model technique. In the latter, analysis of transference and resistance replaces free association as the engine of the treatment. This has a number of consequences, the most far-reaching of which concerns the analyst's behavior. If treatment stands or falls on the analysis of transference, for instance, then analysts must be very careful not to distort or contaminate it. This means that every aspect of their behavior comes under technical pre- and proscriptions. Because Freud was relying on free association and not transference analysis to drive the treatment, he could be much freer in his relations with his patients, as long as he tended sufficiently to their adherence to the fundamental rule.

Thus, in contrast to the basic model technique, Freud's approach is more natural. Analysts speak in a normal voice in a normal manner to their patients. Analysts are not required to hide their beliefs, feelings, and values, though they are free to do so. They need not fear—and patients need not preoccupy themselves with provoking—a personal revelation. Currently, analytic treatment is too often reduced to a cat-and-mouse game between the participants, a game in which the patient tries to catch the analyst in a self-disclosing faux pas and the analyst tries just as desperately to be perfectly invisible—perfect, that is, in an Eisslerian sense. In Freud's approach, the analyst is always fully there, merely acting with a measure of professional restraint and discipline in the service of the task, the discipline being aimed not at being invisible but at noticing counterreactions and taking care that the patient is free-associating.

As the analyst's personality develops and matures across the long sweep of a professional life, it has a natural outlet for expression in Freud's way of working. In the basic model technique, by contrast, analysts strive for abstinence, neutrality, and incognito. If one could achieve this perfect effacement of the self early on, there would be neither need for nor expression of the analyst's personality. One's interpretations would be either right or wrong, and one's communications to patients would remain unchanged in manner from one's 30s to 80s. Presumably, the interpretations would improve, but only in their content, neutrally conveyed, would any expression, however sublimated, occur of the therapist's personality. In the basic model technique the expression of the analyst's maturing personality becomes a parameter.

THE INTERPENETRATION
OF TASK AND METHOD

Freud's definition of the analytic task, to make the unconscious conscious, would be rejected by many analysts today as id psychology. But this task had several important characteristics that made it powerful above and beyond its immediate goal. Most importantly, Freud could rely on a powerful technology with which it was intimately intertwined. When the patient free-associated, the task, more or less dramatically, *was* being accomplished; fresh, unanticipated (by either party) thoughts from the pre- and unconscious parts of the mind came to consciousness and were given voice.

The task in Freud's treatment method also had the advantage of being measurable, clearly defined, and explicit; importantly, it did not burden the treatment with a priori theoretical conceptions about the direction of interpretations and the analysis in general. Freud's definition of the primary task left open the content whereas in some current approaches the direction of the treatment is decided in advance on theoretical grounds. Such preemptive approaches interfere with the emergence of unanticipated material lying outside the domain of the clinician's theory.

Delegating the leadership of the agenda to the patient frees analysts to counterassociate to the material and bend themselves like a receiving organ around the transmitting unconscious of the patient. Within a well-bounded relationship, the elemental structure created by this division of labor frees both parties to think new thoughts. The patient's and analyst's associations make a fertile soil out of which they can collaboratively form unexpected, empirically derived ideas that will be of use to the patient and to the growth of the clinician's knowledge as well.

One gets the impression from formal and informal talks with analytic clinicians that in contemporary treatments the task is often unclear. In general terms, it would be defined as personality change, but this is vague and not easily measured. This vagueness in and of itself does not make the task an unworthy one—patients come to treatment because they want to change, or so they say—but it makes task accomplishment difficult to monitor and consequently brings with it the danger of the task's being displaced by methods that must in a rational enterprise be of only secondary importance. As we have pointed out earlier, the modern insistence on precise and correct procedure can be considered such a displacement of tasks by methods.

One may ask, What is the relationship between making the unconscious conscious and helping patients get better? Has Freud not substituted his own task for the patient's? During his mid-life transition, Freud transformed himself from a neuropsychiatrist to a psychoanalyst and shifted his focus from removing patients' symptoms to enabling them to resume the natural development that comes from living (Newton, 1995). Thus, by about 1900, Freud was becoming less concerned with making his patients healthier or helping them change. Instead, he made sure that they free-associated and told them what he thought was the matter. According to the Wolf Man, Freud said analysis places patients in a position to recover but whether they actually do so depends upon their willpower. With a successful analysis, Freud analogized, one has purchased a train ticket: "This ticket only makes the journey possible; it does not take its place."[1] One of Freud's favorite sayings was, "Je le pansai, Dieu le guérit," meaning that the doctor has to content himself with applying the bandages while some other force, be it God or something in the nature of healing itself—we would say natural, ongoing development—takes care of the rest. Thus, it is true that Freud's definition of the primary task, while full of the wisdom of an experienced, middle-aged clinician, is open to the charge that it may express the doctor's point of view more than the patient's.

OUR DISCOMFORT WITH AUTHORITY

As Lichtenberg and Galler (1987) found, the majority of analysts now avoid directing analysands to free-associate because to do so seems authoritarian and might create a struggle. Here one needs to note again the confusion about authority. Just as there is a problem for a number of modern clinicians in distinguishing between compliance and cooperation, so too is there a related difficulty in distinguishing between being authoritarian and being authoritative. Being authoritarian is to demand compliance to the *principle* of authority. Thus, it is irrational and, as such, has no place in psychoanalytic treatment. Indeed, it is inimical to the task of freeing patients to assume a greater measure of responsibility for themselves. Being authoritative means to represent clearly the requirements of the task in order to enable the patient to cooperate more knowledgeably.

The treatment approach developed by Freud is based on an explicit division of labor about which analyst and analysand, as coworkers, can and should talk, just as colleagues must talk in other forms of work. What is unique to psychoanalysis is that reactions to the inequality of authority not only are free of cost but can be made an important part of the work itself. If the analyst's limited and rational exercise of authority reminds the patient of parental authoritarianism, the analyst should not be misled into imagining that authoritarianism is, in reality, a feature of the treatment. Indeed, the Freudian analyst's explicit use of authority highlights the transference distortion. Too often, with the basic model technique, a situation comes into being that is rarely found outside of contemporary analyses and the novels of Franz Kafka: Neither person is able to speak directly to the other about the reality of their shared situation. The analyst has evoked plenty of transference but has no one to join him or her in trying to understand it. The inability to discuss transference reactions to the clinician's exercise of authority is a powerful stimulus to acting out in both persons. It was this iatrogenically irrational, even destructive, situation that led Ralph Greenson to his strenuous reminders to his colleagues of the importance of the real relationship and the working alliance.

THE DECLINE OF COLLABORATION

Paradoxically, the eschewal that Lichtenberg and Galler (1987) found of the explicit use of authority in psychoanalysis has tended to produce not greater actual equality between clinician and patient but, rather, a steeper tilt to the relationship. The tilt results from the inaccessibility of the analyst and the artificiality of his or her behavior, behavior that is a mystery to the uninitiated and a game, or piece of theater, to the cognoscenti. The increased inequality is manifested concretely in the alteration in the analysand's posture: The patient's torso was upright on Freud's chaise longue, with his or her head at the same level as Freud's, but on the modern flat couch, the analysand is supine, as though on a table, with only a slight elevation of the head. In practice, the more extreme modern tilt in inequality takes apparently opposite forms; the analyst may be either inaccessible or infantilizing.

Eisslerian analysts cannot be spoken to directly, for they are prohibited from engagement. Alexanderian analysts, displaying a unity underlying other differences, do not view the patient as an adult coworker but instead conceive of the treatment in terms of a theory of child development and understand their patients to be children whose treatment experience must be expertly manipulated in the interests of their growth. We hear the latter conception of the patient as adult *manqué* in comments such as "The patient is in the rapprochement subphase; he is practicing" and "The patient needs mirroring" or "She's twenty-eight, but she's *really* three." The task of protecting and rearing small children in the family does require a great inequality in authority; even authoritarian statements such as "You do it because I tell you to do it" may at times be necessary, or at least excusable. But to superimpose this conception of relatedness on the treatment of an adult, even if the treatment is accompanied by generous doses of empathy, warmth, and concern, is inappropriate and, in a strange and unnoticed way, as authoritarian as the basic model technique.

Both the basic model and the remedial child-rearing approaches seem to have as one of their appeals to clinicians an avoidance of the discomfort and embarrassment of exercising authority openly with another adult. More darkly, much modern treatment may provide both parties with a titillating but safe *frisson* of authoritarian sadomasochism, one that for busy middle-class people in a democratic society is hard to come by elsewhere and that neither person is supposed to desire. Were the predilection for keeping authority covert not so ubiquitous, one might suppose that clinicians whose primary experience in the exercise of authority is with children are usually the ones who find this parentalism natural. In reality, authority relations among adults in work are intrinsically troublesome, as we all know from our experiences in the schools, institutes, and clinics in which we work. What is unavoidable in the treatment situation is not just unrealistic conflict, but realistic conflict as well—as we saw in Freud's treatment of Wortis and Kardiner.

Paternal and maternal authoritarianism on the part of the analyst is sometimes justified on the grounds of the patient's low level of development. Yet in his treatment of H.D., who would now be considered borderline, Freud did not lighten the burdens of analysis for her. To the contrary, we find that if the patient has sufficient ego strength to make an expressive psychotherapy feasible, he or she has sufficient ego strength to collaborate responsibly in the treatment. But perhaps in addition to the discomfort with exercising authority directly there is also an economic consideration here: What kind of a living can one make by asking people, especially Americans circa 2000, to be responsible when externalization, acting out, and ego flabbiness may be central to their difficulties?

In Freud's practice, patients were expected to free-associate once they had been shown—repeatedly, if necessary—that they were resisting. Freud treated his patients as novice colleagues who were competent to learn how to assume responsibility for their part of the work in a project significant to both parties. This is what Freud meant when he told Wortis that his continuing to resist interpretations that included criticism of him was purely an emotional reaction that ought to be dropped. By contemporary standards, Freud's statement to Wortis seems utterly absurd. What but purely emotional reactions is the patient supposed to have in psychoanalysis? When we prick a vein, what is the patient to do but bleed? The seeming absurdity to us of Freud's statement tells us how far we have strayed from the conception of analysand as coworker. Freud was acting on his belief that there was more to Wortis than his hurt feelings; that if Wortis tried, he could resume free-associating in spite of them; and that, indeed, if he would only do so, they would very likely learn something new about the hurt feelings rather than continue to be limited to reiterated expressions of petulance. Freud was, in a word, asking Wortis to get back to work. The reader may object, "But, the patient's hurt feelings *were* the work!" Perhaps, but Wortis was not working on them in an effective way. And it is also possible that if he had resumed free-associating, he might have spoken of matters that were quite unpredictably different.

If the analyst has an idea about how the patient should proceed—not the content, but the manner—for the work to be successful, why not tell the patient about it? If the analyst has no such idea, is he or she really competent to undertake the treatment? In reality, most analytic clinicians do have an idea about what constitutes a productive mode of talk from patients but feel they must not express it. The problem with keeping the patient's role obscure is that in failing clearly to tell patients what task achievement requires and helping them learn their part in it, clinicians make it hard for patients to cooperate and remove from them the sense of dignity that comes from learning to be a competent colleague. Moreover, in a situation that stimulates incompetence and childishness, this withholding from the patient of the piece of dignity attendant upon competent work is a painful and superfluous deprivation; there are not many other sources of dignity available in the situation. To overstate the case, it is as though the analyst were saying to the patient, "It is true that I am taking the vestiges of your adulthood from you, but when you have nothing left, you will find me deeply sympathetic."

Analysts ask, "If we direct our patients about how to proceed, won't they simply be submitting to us?" Here we encounter contemporary worries about compliance—as though a compliant attitude could not be confronted and analyzed (as Freud did with the Wolf Man)—and the neglect of cooperation. Indeed, the word "cooperation" seems virtually to have disappeared from analytic discourse. Yet, cooperation was an expression of that part of the transference that was positive and that Freud believed was a *sine qua non* of the treatment.

A PASSIONATE INTEGRATION
OF SCIENCE AND TREATMENT

With the technique of free association, Freud created a method of treatment and research in conformance with a strong predilection of his own. That predilection was evident even in adolescence, when Freud insisted on hearing every aspect of his close friend Eduard Silberstein's experience (Boehlich, 1990). He made the same demands for complete honesty from his fiancée, Martha Bernays, during his 20s (E. Freud, 1960). In his late 30s, Freud became obsessed with finding the childhood secrets that underlay neurosis, even to the point of imagining that every neurotic had been sexually molested. Even after he lost faith in the seduction theory, uncovering hidden truths remained essential in his clinical and scientific work. In an attempt to describe Freud's personality, Jones wrote, "Freud's passion to get at the truth with the maximum of certainty was, I again suggest, the deepest and strongest motive in his nature and the one that impelled him toward his pioneering achievements."[2] This passion for truth characterized his attitude toward man and civilization in general, and his research in particular; it enlivened his clinical procedure as well. In cases as early as that of the Rat Man and as late as that of H.D., his patients, too, can be seen to be swept up in the excitement of discovery. The Wolf Man wrote of his treatment, "In my analysis with Freud I felt myself less as a patient than as a co-worker, the younger comrade of an experienced explorer setting out to study a new, recently discovered land."[3]

Freud's work was dedicated to unraveling unconscious meaning, and he enlisted his patients' active help in this endeavor. He could be unrelenting in this search and blunt about his findings. To his patients this could be painful as well as inspiring, but most were impressed with the intensity of Freud's commitment to the task. Blanton said at the end of his analysis, "I think a great deal of the benefit I have had from my analysis is the association with you and the appreciation of your courage, your scientific manner, and your sympathy."[4] Freud expected the same dedication from his patients. In the interest of extending the control of conscious reasoning over the powers of the unconscious and thus freeing themselves from its influence, patients were expected to adopt a scientific attitude toward their own treatment.

Freud understood that this was not easily done, but he never promised easy cures. He always emphasized that psychoanalysis requires sacrifices and that suffering is intrinsic to the work. Therefore, patients like Wortis, whose entire defensive system was mobilized against the realization that something might be the matter with him, did not fare well with Freud. As Wortis frequently pointed out, to the extent that Freud demanded compliance, it was with respect to the task, which became the very focus of Wortis's manifest resistance. Freud criticized Wortis for not having a scientific attitude and told him repeatedly that his interpretations, no matter how painful their content, were not made for personal reasons but for the sake of the treatment and the truth.

Freud's efforts with Wortis were wasted (at least Wortis did not indicate otherwise), but other patients responded more favorably to his passion, even if they were sometimes roughed up by his interpretations. The value of his attitude ultimately transcended the level of the personal, even if that is where it found its most immediate expression. Thus, it is misleading to say that Freud's technique derived its power solely from his personality. First of all, he had a technique to which he devoted himself; second, his personality was subordinated to the pursuit of greater ideals, as his patients well knew. Freud had remarkable sublimatory powers; his capacity to transform instinctual drives into cultural aims, a phenomenon always mysterious, now seems to us almost a piece of lost magic from a distant time. Freud's way of doing analysis naturally included his passion for the truth.

Freud was more interested in the id and its contents than the ego and its defenses. Even though his theory about the importance of resistances and unconscious defense mechanisms had already been in place for a long time when he began treating the patients whose cases are examined in this book, he did not work with these patients in ways now recommended. Freud could be demanding of his patients and expected them to mobilize the healthy parts of their egos for the work. The positive transference helped to make this possible. While he could be reproached for neglecting to analyze the sick parts consistently, Freud also did not support the regressive trends in his patients. By addressing himself to the healthy or mature aspects of his patients' ego, he treated them as adults capable of putting immediate impulses or wishes for gratification aside in the interest of achieving a higher level of personality organization.

Freud's belief in the ability of patients, aided by the positive transference, to rally and commit themselves to the work in defiance of regressive intoxifications would today be considered by many to be unanalytic. The same is true of his commitment to the idea that increased knowledge brings substantial therapeutic gain. Freud struggled with the significance of conscious knowledge for successful psychoanalytic treatment, alternately attributing importance to it and rejecting it. In most of the cases reviewed in this book, knowledge and insight played an important role. Freud's belief in willpower based on rationality—which, as Kardiner learned, was all there was to his notion of working through—in opposition to some of his other ideas concerning resistance and the death instinct, shows his intellectual attachment to the values and ethos of the European Enlightenment. A half century after Freud, the belief that reason will triumph over irrationality is hard for us to sustain, although we should note that it was not easy in Freud's time, either. The attempt to be reasonable, psychoanalytically expanded to include the greatest possible felt knowledge of the irrational and its ubiquity, remains an ideal that is useful in treatment, as well as in living and in research, one capable of sustaining and enhancing life for both patient and clinician. It did so for Freud and for most of the patients who wrote about their encounters with him.

Notes

INTRODUCTION

1. Cremerius (1981, p. 147).
2. Ibid.
3. Momigliano (1987, p. 387).
4. Ellman (1991, p. 286).
5. Wortis (1954, p. 73).
6. Miller and Rice (1967, p. 4).

CHAPTER ONE

1. Jones (1955, p. 230).
2. Apparently, Freud had written some 50 pages for the textbook before giving up on it. Jones (1955) wrote, "Nothing more was heard of the project, nor have those precious pages been preserved. 'Suddenly, as rare things will, it vanished' " (p. 231).
3. Coltrera and Ross (1967, p. 39).
4. Freud (1905a, pp. 257–258).
5. Roazen (1975, p. 118).
6. Jones (1955, p. 233).
7. Freud (1910c, p. 226).
8. Fenichel (1938–1939, p. 1).
9. Freud (1913a, p. 123).
10. Ibid.
11. Freud (1913a, p. 123; 1913b, p. 183).
12. Freud (1913a, p. 125).
13. Freud (1912c, p. 111).

14. Jones (1955, p. 241).
15. Ibid.
16. Freud (1910c, p. 226).
17. Ferenczi (1928, p. 89).
18. Freud (1914a, p. 155).
19. Freud (1910c, p. 225).
20. Gray (1994, p. 35).
21. Ibid., p. 37.
22. Freud (1913a, p. 141).
23. Freud (1910c, p. 226).
24. Freud (1914a, p. 154).
25. Freud (1912c, p. 118).
26. Freud (1912a, p. 108).
27. Freud (1913a, p. 139).
28. Freud (1912c, p. 115).
29. Ibid., p. 111.
30. Ibid., p. 112.
31. A term Freud (1912c, p. 116) attributed to Stekel.
32. Freud (1913a, p. 140).
33. Freud (1912c, p. 115).
34. Freud (1912c, p. 116).
35. Freud (1911a, p. 94).
36. Ibid.
37. Ibid., p. 92.
38. Some critics, for instance, explain Freud's clinical behavior as being the result of arbitrariness and, essentially, narcissism; in other words, they reproach him for not following his own teachings because he felt himself to be exempt from such rules.

CHAPTER TWO

1. Frink was in analysis with Freud from March 1920 to June 1921 (Jones, 1957, p. 85).
2. Kardiner (1977, p. 15). Freud was accumulating foreign currency at the time to prevent another financial crisis like the one he and other Austrians experienced following the collapse of the Austrian currency immediately after World War I (Jones, 1957, p. 29).
3. From Jones (1957, p. 88) we know that Freud, trying to accommodate the increasing number of analysands from abroad, found it difficult to conduct several hours of treatment a day in English; it left him "drained."
4. After the difficulties of the war years, Freud was now very busy in his private practice. From this time on he accepted more pupils than patients (Jones, 1957, p. 78).
5. Kardiner (1977, p. 17).
6. In a letter to Ferenczi, Freud wrote that he had promised to analyze twice as

many people as he could actually manage. He eventually took on ten (Jones, 1957, p. 78).

7. Kardiner, 1977, p. 18.
8. Ibid., p. 23.
9. Ibid., p. 42.
10. Ibid., p. 37.
11. Ibid., p. 51.
12. Ibid., p. 55.
13. Ibid., p. 56.
14. Ibid.
15. Ibid., p. 57.
16. Ibid., p. 58.
17. Ibid.
18. Ibid., p. 60.
19. Ibid., p. 61.
20. Ibid.
21. Ibid., p. 67. Since his analysis with Freud in 1921, Frink had become involved in a scandal. He had fallen in love with a patient and wanted to marry her. Both needed to obtain a divorce first, but the patient's husband caused a furor. The analytic community was up in arms. According to Jones, Freud supported Frink's plan (Jones, 1957, p. 85).
22. Kardiner (1977, p. 62).
23. Ibid., p. 63.
24. Ibid., p. 68.
25. Ibid.
26. Ibid., p. 75.
27. Ibid., p. 76.
28. Ibid., p. 77.
29. Ibid., p. 74.
30. Ibid., p. 78.
31. Ibid., p. 69.
32. Ibid., p. 11.

CHAPTER THREE

1. Doolittle (*Correspondence with Bryher MacPherson*, March 21, 1933). This correspondence is as yet unpublished. Permission to quote was obtained from the Yale Beinecke Rare Book and Manuscript Library.
2. Sachs could not continue with the analysis because he was moving to the United States. He helped her chances of being accepted for analysis with Freud by writing a letter of introduction.
3. H.D. (*Correspondence*, March 1, 1933).
4. Ibid.
5. Ibid.
6. Ibid.

7. H.D. saw Freud six times a week in 1933 and five times a week in 1934.
8. H.D. (1956, p. 69).
9. Ibid., pp. 119–120.
10. Bryher, a wealthy woman and ardent supporter of psychoanalysis, had been instrumental in getting H.D. into treatment, first with Sachs and Chadwick and then Freud. She not only paid for H.D.'s analysis but made large financial contributions to the psychoanalytic society as well.
11. H.D. paid $25 an hour in 1934 and a little less in 1933.
12. H.D. (*Correspondence*, March 4, 1933).
13. Case (1989, p. 102).
14. H.D. (1956, p. 129).
15. Ibid., p. 130.
16. H.D. (*Correspondence*, March 6, 1933).
17. Ibid., March 18, 1933.
18. H.D. (1956, p. 136).
19. Ibid., p. 139.
20. Ibid., pp. 14–16.
21. H.D. (*Correspondence*, March 9, 1933).
22. H.D. (1956, p. 152).
23. H.D. (*Correspondence*, March 10, 1933).
24. H.D. (1956, p. 148).
25. Ibid., p. 150.
26. Ibid., p. 152.
27. Van Eck is the pseudonym used in H.D.'s *Tribute to Freud*. In the correspondence this man is referred to as Rodeck.
28. H.D. (1956, p. 161).
29. Ibid., pp. 163–164.
30. Ibid.
31. H.D. (*Correspondence*, March 16, 1933).
32. H.D. (1956, p. 168).
33. Ibid.
34. Ibid., pp. 55–56.
35. Ibid., p. 171.
36. H.D. (*Correspondence*, March 18, 1933).
37. H.D. (1956, p. 173).
38. Ibid.
39. Ibid., p. 175.
40. H.D. (*Correspondence*, March 21, 1933).
41. Freud discussed this theory in his 1931 paper "Female Sexuality."
42. H.D. (1956, p. 176).
43. H.D. (*Correspondence*, March 23, 1933).
44. H.D. (1956, p. 177).
45. Ibid., p. 181.
46. Ibid.
47. Ibid., p. 184.
48. H.D. (*Correspondence*, March 25, 1933).
49. Ibid.

50. Ibid.
51. Ibid., April 17, 1933.
52. Ibid., April 21, 1933.
53. Ibid., April 22, 1933.
54. Ibid., April 25, 1933.
55. Ibid., April 27, 1933.
56. Ibid.
57. Ibid.
58. Ibid., April 28, 1933.
59. Ibid., April 24 or 25, 1933.
60. Ibid.
61. Ibid., April 28, 1933.
62. Ibid.
63. Ibid., April 30, 1933.
64. H.D. (1956, pp. 61–62).
65. H.D. (*Correspondence*, May 3, 1933).
66. Ibid., May 6, 1933.
67. Ibid., May 7, 1933.
68. Ibid., May 9, 1933.
69. Ibid., May 15, 1933.
70. Ibid., May 17, 1933.
71. Ibid., May 18, 1933.
72. Ibid.
73. Ibid., May 21, 1933.
74. Ibid., May 23, 1933.
75. Ibid., May 26, 1933.
76. Ibid.
77. Ibid.
78. Ibid., May 28, 1933.
79. Ibid.
80. H.D. (1956, p. 6).
81. H.D. (*Correspondence*, November 7, 1934).
82. Ibid., November 8, 1934.
83. Ibid., November 11, 1934.
84. Ibid., November 14, 1934.
85. Ibid., November 15, 1934.
86. Ibid., November 16, 1934.
87. Ibid., November 19, 1934.
88. Ibid.
89. Ibid., November 22, 1934.
90. Ibid., November 24, 1934.
91. Ibid., November 27, 1934.
92. Ibid., November 29, 1934. The particular puppy they were supposed to have taken turned out to be wild and destructive. He had to be put to sleep by his new owners.
93. Ibid., December 2, 1934.

CHAPTER FOUR

1. Wortis (1954, p. 8).
2. Ibid., p. 9.
3. Ibid., p. 5.
4. Ibid., p. 10.
5. Ibid., p. 12.
6. Ibid., p. 13.
7. Ibid., p. 15.
8. At five meetings a week, this would come to a fee of $20 per session, which was slightly less than H.D.'s $25 fee in 1934.
9. Wortis (1954, p. 16).
10. Ibid.
11. Ibid., p. 17.
12. Ibid.
13. Ibid.
14. Ibid., p. 19.
15. Ibid., pp. 20–21.
16. Ibid., p. 22.
17. Ibid.
18. Ibid., p. 24.
19. Ibid., p. 26.
20. Ibid.
21. Ibid., p. 27.
22. Ibid., p. 28.
23. Ibid., p. 29.
24. Ibid., p. 30.
25. Stekel was one of Freud's oldest disciples. Freud had made Stekel and Adler editors of the *Zentralblatt* in 1910. His difficulties with Stekel were not about psychoanalytic theory, as had been the case with Adler. Even though Freud valued Stekel's contribution to the understanding of symbolism, he found him dishonest and his methods unscientific; he once referred to him as a case of "moral insanity" (Jones, 1955, p. 137). Their strained relationship came to an end in 1912 over an argument involving Tausk.
26. Wortis (1954, p. 31).
27. Ibid., p. 32.
28. Ibid., p. 33.
29. Ibid., p. 35.
30. Ibid., p. 36.
31. Ibid., p. 37.
32. Ibid., p. 39.
33. Ibid.
34. Ibid., p. 40.
35. Ibid., p. 41.
36. Ibid.
37. Ibid.

38. Ibid. Magnus Hirschfeld was a sexologist who had at one point belonged to the Psychoanalytic Society in Berlin, founded by Karl Abraham in 1908. However, according to Gay (1988), he was interested in sexual liberation, not psychoanalysis, and dropped out.
39. Ibid., p. 43.
40. Ibid., p. 44.
41. Ibid.
42. Ibid., p. 45.
43. Ibid.
44. Ibid., p. 47.
45. Ibid., p. 48.
46. Ibid.
47. Ibid., p. 49.
48. Ibid., p. 59.
49. Ibid., p. 50.
50. Ibid., p. 51.
51. Ibid., p. 57.
52. Ibid.
53. Ibid., p. 58.
54. Ibid., p. 60.
55. Ibid., p. 61.
56. Ibid., p. 62.
57. Ibid.
58. Ibid., p. 64.
59. Ibid., p. 69.
60. Ibid., p. 71.
61. Ibid., p. 73.
62. Ibid., p. 76.
63. Ibid.
64. Ibid., p. 77.
65. Ibid., p. 79.
66. Ibid., p. 81.
67. Ibid.
68. Ibid., p. 82.
69. Ibid., p. 83.
70. Ibid., p. 86.
71. Ibid., p. 89.
72. Ibid., p. 92.
73. Ibid., p. 94.
74. Ibid., p. 95.
75. Ibid., p. 96.
76. Ibid., p. 110.
77. Ibid., p. 112.
78. Ibid., pp. 114–115.
79. Ibid., p. 117.
80. Ibid., p. 120.
81. Ibid., p. 128.

82. Ibid., p. 129.
83. Ibid., p. 136.
84. Ibid., p. 137.
85. Ibid., p. 143.
86. Ibid., p. 153.
87. Ibid., p. 156.
88. Wortis later added to his notes that Freud must have heard the information about Ellis's wife being homosexual from someone else; Ellis's autobiography, published subsequently, actually supports this hypothesis. Wortis could not know that H.D. had talked to Freud about her intimate relationship with Ellis in detail; she might have been the source of this information.
89. Wortis (1954, p. 162).
90. Ibid.

CHAPTER FIVE

1. Dorsey (1976, p. 16).
2. Ibid., p. 19.
3. Dorsey's analysis was paid for by the Rockefeller grant financing his sabbatical leave.
4. Ibid., p. 20.
5. Ibid., pp. 21, 46.
6. Ibid., p. 23.
7. Ibid., p. 49.
8. Ibid., p. 26.
9. Ibid.
10. Ibid., p. 27.
11. Ibid., p. 53.
12. Ibid., p. 9.
13. Ibid., p. 65.
14. Ibid., p. 60.
15. Ibid., p. 29.
16. Ibid., p. 24.
17. Ibid., p. 42.
18. Ibid., p. 69.
19. Ibid., p. 43.
20. Ibid., p. 26.
21. Ibid., p. 32.
22. Ibid., p. 35.
23. Ibid., p. 43.
24. Ibid., p. 36.
25. Ibid.
26. Ibid., p. 74.
27. Ibid., p. 132.
28. Ibid., p. 60.

29. Ibid., p. xv.
30. Ibid., p. 35.
31. Ibid., p. 37.
32. Ibid., p. 48.
33. Ibid.
34. Ibid., p. 71.
35. Ibid., p. 34.
36. Ibid., p. 66.
37. Ibid., p. 68.
38. Ibid., p. 73.
39. Ibid., p. 62.
40. Ibid., p. 78.
41. Ibid.
42. Ibid., p. 101.
43. Ibid., p. x.
44. Ibid., p. 131.
45. Ibid.

CHAPTER SIX

1. Blanton (1971, p. 20).
2. Ibid., p. 21.
3. Blanton's history is not included in his journal notes. His wife added it in an addendum.
4. Blanton (1971, p. 121).
5. Ibid., p. 21.
6. Ibid., p. 22.
7. Ibid., p. 23.
8. Ibid., p. 27.
9. Ibid.
10. Ibid.
11. Ibid., p. 28.
12. Ibid., pp. 29–30.
13. Ibid.
14. Ibid., p. 31.
15. Ibid., p. 32.
16. Ibid.
17. Ibid., pp. 34–35.
18. Ibid., p. 36.
19. Ibid.
20. Ibid., p. 37.
21. Ibid., p. 41.
22. Ibid., p. 42.
23. Ibid., p. 44.
24. Ibid., p. 45.

25. Ibid., p. 46.
26. Ibid., p. 47.
27. Ibid., p. 48.
28. Ibid.
29. Ibid., p. 52.
30. As we have seen in his treatment of H.D., Freud was still working on this idea four years later.
31. Blanton (1971, p. 54).
32. Unfortunately, Blanton's wife deleted many of the dreams from the published version of the journal. She thought they were too personal in nature and difficult to understand out of context.
33. Blanton (1971, p. 56).
34. Ibid.
35. Ibid.
36. Ibid., pp. 57–58.
37. Ibid., p. 59.
38. Ibid., p. 61.
39. Ibid., p. 62.
40. Ibid., pp. 64–65.
41. Ibid., p. 65.
42. Ibid.
43. Ibid., pp. 65–66.
44. Ibid., p. 67.
45. Ibid., p. 68.
46. Ibid.
47. Ibid., pp. 68–69.
48. Ibid., p. 69.
49. Ibid., pp. 70–71.
50. Ibid., p. 76.
51. Ibid.
52. Ibid., p. 78.
53. Ibid.
54. Ibid., p. 79.
55. Ibid., pp. 80–81.
56. Ibid., p. 81.
57. Ibid., p. 84.
58. Ibid.
59. Ibid., p. 86.
60. Ibid., p. 88.
61. Ibid., p. 90.
62. Ibid.
63. Ibid., p. 91.
64. Ibid., p. 92.
65. Ibid.
66. Ibid., p. 96.
67. Ibid., p. 98.
68. Ibid., p. 100.

69. Ibid., p. 102.
70. Ibid.
71. Ibid.
72. Ibid.
73. Ibid., p. 103.
74. Ibid., p. 106.
75. Ibid., p. 111.
76. Ibid., p. 112.
77. Ibid., p. 113.
78. Ibid., p. 115.
79. Ibid., p. 117.
80. Ibid., p. 118.

CHAPTER SEVEN

1. H.D. (1956, p. 16).
2. Riviere (1939, p. 129).
3. Wortis (1954, p. 64).
4. H.D. (*Correspondence*, November 7, 1934).
5. H.D. (1956, p. 18).
6. Ibid., p. 177.
7. Blanton (1971, p. 28).
8. Ibid., pp. 75–76.
9. Kardiner (1977, p. 58).
10. H.D. (1956, p. 18).
11. Freud (1940a, p. 173).
12. Ibid.
13. Money-Kyrle (1979, p. 267).
14. H.D. (1956, p. 162).
15. H.D. (*Correspondence*, May 3, 1933).
16. Gray (1994, p. 37).
17. Freud (1940a, p. 174).
18. H.D. (1956, p. 125).
19. Freud thought he had found "the solution of a more-than-thousand-year-old problem, a caput Nili [source of the Nile]," with the theory that childhood seduction lay at the root of hysteria (Masson, 1985, p. 184; Schröter, 1986, p. 193).
20. Khan (1973, p. 370).
21. H.D. (1956, p. 22).
22. Kardiner (1977, p. 57).
23. Choisy (1963, p. 7).
24. Wortis (1954, p. 61).
25. Dorsey (1976, p. 36).
26. H.D. (1956, p. 116).
27. Ibid., p. viii.

28. H.D. (*Correspondence*, May 3, 1933).
29. Ruitenbeek (1973, p. 359).
30. H.D. (1956, pp. 163, 171).
31. H.D. (*Correspondence*, May 18, 1933).
32. Ibid., November 27, 1934.
33. Kardiner (1977, p. 68).
34. Blanton (1971, p. 76).
35. Ibid., pp. 34–35.
36. Wortis (1954, p. 20).
37. Blanton (1971, p. 23).
38. Ibid., pp. 36, 54.
39. Wortis (1954, p. 71).
40. Dorsey (1976, p. 29).
41. Ibid., p. 38.
42. Ibid., p. 43.
43. Blanton (1971, p. 68).
44. Newton (1995, p. 138 and p. 138, n. 87).
45. Freud (1925, p. 40).
46. Ibid., p. 42.
47. Ibid., p. 41.
48. Freud (1925) compared interpretation to free association and called it a "related art" (p. 43).
49. Wortis (1954, pp. 126–127).
50. Freud (1925, p. 40).
51. Wortis (1954, p. 26).
52. H.D. (*Correspondence*, March 23, 1933).
53. Freud (1940a, p. 173).
54. H.D. (*Correspondence*, March 25, 1933).
55. Freud (1914a, p. 155).
56. Blanton (1971, p. 54).
57. Wortis (1954, p. 43).
58. Ibid., pp. 43, 143.
59. Blanton (1971, p. 32).
60. Wortis (1954, p. 43).
61. Riviere (1939, pp. 129–130).
62. H.D. (1956, p. 171).
63. Riviere (1939, p. 129.
64. Wortis (1954, p. 153).
65. Freud (1916–1917, p. 83; 1940, p. 172).
66. Wortis (1954, p. 82).
67. Blanton (1971, p. 46).
68. Wortis (1954, p. 82).
69. Ibid., pp. 82, 40, 85, 95, 125.
70. Blanton (1971, p. 30).
71. Kardiner (1977, p. 57).
72. Choisy (1963, p. 6).
73. Ibid., p. 7.

74. Bertin (1982, p. 160).
75. Newton (1995, p. 190).
76. Ibid, pp. 207–209.
77. Freud (1925, p. 43).
78. Jones (1953, p. 353).
79. Freud (1900, p. 133).
80. Ibid., p. 194; Masson (1985, p. 270). See also Schröter (1986, p. 296 and p. 296, n. 3).
81. Masson (1985, p. 274).
82. Freud (1940a, p. 179).
83. Freud (1914a, p. 155).
84. Freud (1914b, pp. 214–215). Freud uses the terms *Überwindung* ("overcoming"), *Widerstand aufdecken* ("uncover"), *Widerstand benennen* ("naming"), *sich in den Widerstand vertiefen* ("to become absorbed in or deepen"), and *Widerstand durcharbeiten* ("working through").
85. Ibid., p. 215.
86. Wortis (1954, p. 49).
87. Ibid., p. 139.
88. Blanton (1971, p. 68).
89. Dorsey (1976, pp. 65, 24).
90. Freud (1925, p. 41).
91. Wortis (1954, p. 24).
92. H.D. (*Correspondence*, November 22, 1934).
93. Blanton (1971, p. 69).
94. Wortis (1954, p. 70).
95. H.D. (*Correspondence*, March 25, 1933).
96. Ibid., November 11, 1934.
97. Blanton (1971, p. 29).
98. Ibid., p. 42.
99. H.D. (*Correspondence*, November 22, 1934).
100. H.D. (1956, p. 184).
101. H.D. (*Correspondence*, November 1, 1934).
102. Wortis (1954, p. 61).
103. Blanton (1971, p. 69).
104. H.D. (*Correspondence*, March 9, 1933).
105. Blanton (1971, p. 32).
106. H.D. (*Correspondence*, March 25, 1933).
107. H.D. (1956, p. 17).
108. Wortis (1954, p. 58).
109. Ibid., p. 89.
110. Ibid., p. 96.
111. Ibid., p. 64.
112. Freud (1914a, p. 154).
113. Freud (1925, p. 42).
114. Dorsey (1976, p. 62).
115. Wortis (1954, p. 82).
116. Ibid., p. 137.

117. Blanton (1971, pp. 68, 103).
118. Deutsch (1973, p. 133).
119. Money-Kyrle (1979, p. 267).
120. Freud (1925, pp. 42–43).
121. In Ruitenbeek (1973, p. 359).
122. Freud (1925, p. 42).
123. Wortis (1954, p. 112).
124. H.D. (*Correspondence*, March 1, 1933).
125. Freud (1925, p. 43).
126. Wortis (1954, pp. 48, 78, 112).
127. Money-Kyrle (1979, p. 267).
128. H.D. (1956, p. 147). In a similar vein, Freud told Kardiner that he was too much the father to be a good therapist (Kardiner, 1977, p. 69).
129. Freud (1905a, p. 259).
130. Wortis (1954, p. 73).
131. Blanton (1971, pp. 21, 22).
132. Ibid., p. 65.
133. H.D. (1956, p. 175).

CHAPTER EIGHT

1. For a fascinating discussion on the effects of transplanting European ideas, including psychoanalysis, to the United States in the 20th century, see H. Stuart Hughes (1975), *The Sea Change*.
2. Haynal (1989) refers to classical technique after Freud as "post-classical" to distinguish between the two; Lipton (1977) refers to "modern technique" and reserves the term "classical technique" for Freud's method.
3. This shift from analytic task to behavior is illustrated, for example, by the modern concern with what Lipton (1977) calls "trivial matters" (p. 262), such as the fact that the Rat Man spent several sessions sitting up or walking around rather than lying on the couch.
4. Ibid.
5. Freud to Ferenczi (1928), quoted in Jones (1955, p. 241).
6. Eissler (1953, p. 105).
7. Ibid., p. 125.
8. Eissler (1953, p. 120) takes the term "ego modification" from Riviere's translation of Freud's "Analysis Terminable and Interminable" (1937a). Freud's original term was *Ichveränderung*.
9. Ibid., p. 122.
10. Ibid., p. 108.
11. Lipton (1977, p. 264).
12. Eissler (1953, p. 110).
13. Ibid., p. 126.
14. See also Kanzer and Blum (1967): "Adherence to the fundamental rule in the analytic setting has as its complement a basically self-effacing position of the analyst" (p. 104).

15. Eissler (1958, pp. 222–223), quoted in Valenstein (1979, p. 117).
16. Wallerstein (1995, p. 111).
17. See, for example, Kanzer and Blum (1967): "We agree with the position generally taken, that, in the end, analytic technique depends on the clinical experiences of the practitioner and on his personal analysis and individual training" (p. 328). Also Greenson, quoted in Kanzer (1979): "Much subjectivity exists in the exercise of a 'lonely profession . . . [where] the analyst's own view of what he does is unreliable and apt to be distorted in some idealized direction' " (p. 338).
18. Gay (1988, p. 499).
19. Freud (1926a, p. 248).
20. Gray (1994, pp. 49, 54).
21. Ibid., pp. 54, 52.
22. Eissler (1963, p. 106).
23. Lipton (1977, p. 263).
24. Stone (1961, pp. 28, 30).
25. Eissler (1958, pp. 223, 228–229).
26. Nacht (1958, p. 235).
27. Ibid., p. 236.
28. Stone (1961, p. 19).
29. Freud (1940a, p. 177).
30. Stone (1961, p. 33).
31. Ibid., p. 28.
32. Freud (1915a, p. 165).
33. Freud (1919a, p. 162).
34. Ibid., p. 164.
35. Ibid.
36. Stone (1961, p. 23).
37. Freud (1912c, p. 115).
38. Naive therapeutic ambitiousness had gotten Freud, then in his 20s, into trouble with his friend Ernst von Fleischl-Marxow, for whom he prescribed cocaine. It led him in his 30s to the nearly disastrous referral of his patient Emma Eckstein to his colleague Wilhelm Fliess for a nose operation. It was responsible for a more enduring tendency on Freud's part to tell patients, as he did with Dora when he was in his 40s, things about themselves that they were not ready to hear.
39. Stone (1961, p. 26).
40. Freud (1912c, p. 118).
41. Stone (1961, p. 27).
42. Freud (1915b, p. 224).
43. Freud (1915a, p. 164; 1915b, p. 224).
44. Freud (1915a, p. 170).
45. Freud (1915b, p. 229).
46. Stone (1961, p. 28).
47. Greenson (1967, p. 220).
48. Lipton (1977, p. 268).
49. Freud (1909a, p. 159).

50. Ibid., p. 166.
51. Ibid.
52. Gray (1994, p. 47).
53. Freud (1912c, p. 114).
54. Zetzel (1966, p. 129).
55. Ibid., p. 128.
56. Bergmann and Hartman (1976, p. 164).
57. Langs (1980, p. 215).
58. Ibid., pp. 215–216.
59. The language of "violations" is odd and has contributed to Langs's isolation within psychoanalysis. How could a frame be *violated?* The imagery is confused, violent, and moralistic. It is one thing to say, as both Langs and Newton (1971, 1973a, 1989, 1992) have, that the structure and boundaries of the treatment system are important; it is quite another to say that in making or allowing changes in them, the clinician is violating the patient.
60. Holland (1969, p. 315).
61. Freud (1918). We have approximated the patient's age from the material on pp. 7–8.
62. Ibid., p. 11.
63. Ibid.
64. Ibid., p. 76.
65. Gedo and Goldberg (1973, p. 260).
66. Freud (1918, p. 11).
67. Weiss (1980, p. 213).

CHAPTER NINE

1. Newton (1995, p. 148).
2. Jones (1955, p. 433).
3. "My Recollections of Sigmund Freud," by the Wolf-Man. In Gardiner (1971, p. 140).
4. Blanton (1971, p. 112).

References

Alexander, F., & French, T. M. (1946). *Psychoanalytic Therapy: Principles and Applications*. New York: Ronald Press.

Bergmann, M., & Hartman, F. (Eds.). (1976). *The Evolution of Psychoanalytic Technique*. New York: Basic Books.

Bertin, C. (1982). *Marie Bonaparte: A Life*. New Haven, CT: Yale University Press.

Bettelheim, B. (1982). *Freud and Man's Soul*. New York: Random House.

Blanton, S. (1971). *Diary of My Analysis with Sigmund Freud*. New York: Hawthorn Books.

Boehlich, W. (Ed.). (1990). *The Letters of Sigmund Freud to Eduard Silberstein, 1871–1881*. Cambridge, MA: Harvard University Press.

Bräutigam, W. (1983). "Beziehung und Übertragung in Freud's Behandlungen und Schriften [Relationship and Transference in Freud's Cases and Papers]." *Psyche, 37*(2): 116–129.

Case, L. (1989). *H.D. and Her Poetry: An Adult Developmental Study*. Unpublished doctoral dissertation, The Wright Institute, Berkeley, CA.

Choisy, M. (1963). *Sigmund Freud: A New Appraisal*. New York: Citadel Press.

Coltrera, J., & Ross, N. (1967). "Freud's Psychoanalytic Technique: From the Beginnings to 1923." In B. B. Wolman (Ed.), *Psychoanalytic Techniques: A Handbook for the Practicing Psychoanalyst*. New York: Basic Books.

Cremerius, J. (1981). "Freud bei der Arbeit über die Schulter Geschaut: Seine Technik im Spiegel von Schülern und Patienten [Freud at Work: His Technique in the Mirror of Students and Patients]." *Jahrbuch der Psychoanalyse*, Vol. 6. Bern: Hans Huber.

De Saussure, R. (1956). "Sigmund Freud." In H. M. Ruitenbeek (Ed.), *Freud As We Knew Him*. Detroit: Wayne State University Press, 1973.

Deutsch, H. (1973). *Confrontations with Myself: An Epilogue*. New York: Norton.

Doolittle, H. (1956). *Tribute to Freud*. New York: New Directions.

————. (1988). *Correspondence with Bryher MacPherson*. Previously unpublished material by H.D. (Hilda Doolittle).

Dorsey, J. M. (1976). *An American Psychiatrist in Vienna, 1935–1937, and His Sigmund Freud*. Detroit: Center for Health Education.

————. (1980). *University Professor John Dorsey*. Detroit: Wayne State University Press.

Eagle, J., & Newton, P. (1981). "Scapegoating in Small Groups: An Organizational Approach." *Human Relations, 34*(4): 283–301.

Eissler, K. R. (1950). "The Chicago Institute of Psychoanalysis and the Sixth Period of the Development of Psychoanalytic Technique." *Journal of General Psychology, 42*: 103–157.

————. (1953). "The Effect of the Structure of the Ego on Psychoanalytic Technique." *Journal of the American Psychoanalytic Association, 1*: 104–143.

————. (1958). "Remarks on Some Variations in Psycho-Analytical Technique." *International Journal of Psycho-Analysis, 39*: 222–229.

Ellman, S. (1991). *Freud's Technique Papers: A Contemporary Perspective*. Northvale, NJ: Aronson.

Faber, M. D. (1970). "Allport's Visit with Freud." *Psychoanalytic Review, 57*(1): 60–64.

Fenichel, O. (1938–1939). *Problems of Psychoanalytic Technique* (D. Brunswick, Trans.). Albany: Psychoanalytic Quarterly, 1941.

————. (1945). *The Psychoanalytic Theory of Neurosis*. New York: Norton.

Ferenczi, S. (1919). "Technical Difficulties in the Analysis of a Case of Hysteria" (J. Suttie, Trans.). In E. Jones (Ed.), *Further Contributions to the Theory and Technique of Psychoanalysis* (2nd ed.). London: Hogarth Press and the Institute of Psycho-Analysis, 1950.

————. (1928). "The Elasticity of Psycho-Analytic Technique." In *Final Contributions to the Problems and Methods of Psycho-Analysis*. London: Hogarth Press, 1955.

————, & Rank, O. (1924). *The Development of Psycho-Analysis*. New York and Washington: Nervous and Mental Disease Publishing Co.

Freud, E. L. (Ed.). (1960). *Letters of Sigmund Freud*. New York: Basic Books.

Freud, S. (1895). *Studies on Hysteria*. In J. Strachey (Ed. and Trans.), *The Standard Edition of the Complete Psychological Works of Sigmund Freud* (Vol. 2). London: Hogarth Press, 1955.

————. (1896). "Heredity and the Aetiology of the Neuroses." *SE*, Vol. 3, 1962: 143–156.

————. (1900). *The Interpretation of Dreams*. *SE*, Vols. 4 & 5, 1953.

————. (1904). "Freud's Psycho-Analytic Procedure." *SE*, Vol. 7, 1953: 249–254.

————. (1905a). "On Psychotherapy." *SE*, Vol. 7, 1953: 257–268.

————. (1905b). "Über Psychotherapie." In A. Mitscherlich, A. Richards, & J. Strachey (Eds.), *Sigmund Freud: Schriften zur Behandlungstechnik. Studienausgabe* (Ergänzungsband). Frankfurt am Rhein: Fischer, 1982: 107–119.

————. (1905c). "Fragment of an Analysis of a Case of Hysteria." *SE*, Vol. 7, 1953: 7–122.

————. (1909a). *Notes upon a Case of Obsessional Neurosis*. *SE*, Vol. 10, 1955: 155–318.

_____. (1909b). "Analysis of a Phobia in a Five-Year-Old Boy." *SE*, Vol. 10, 1955: 5–149.

_____. (1910a). "The Future Prospects of Psycho-Analytic Therapy." *SE*, Vol. 11, 1957: 139–153.

_____. (1910b). "Die zukünftigen Chancen der Psychoanalytischen Therapie." *Studienausgabe*: 121–132.

_____. (1910c). " 'Wild' Psycho-Analysis." *SE*, Vol. 11, 1957: 221–227.

_____. (1910d). "Über 'wilde' Psychoanalyse." *Studienausgabe*: 133–141.

_____. (1911a). "The Handling of Dream-Interpretation in Psycho-Analysis." *SE*, Vol. 12, 1958: 91–96.

_____. (1911b). "Die Handhabung der Traumdeutung in der Psychoanalyse." *Studienausgabe*: 149–156.

_____. (1912a). "The Dynamics of Transference." *SE*, Vol. 12, 1958: 99–108.

_____. (1912b). "Zur Dynamik der Übertragung." *Studienausgabe*: 157–168.

_____. (1912c). "Recommendations to Physicians Practising Psycho-Analysis." *SE*, Vol. 12, 1958: 111–120.

_____. (1912d). "Ratschläge für den Arzt bei der psychoanalytischen Behandlung." *Studienausgabe*: 169–180.

_____. (1913a). "On Beginning the Treatment (Further Recommendations on the Technique of Psycho-Analysis I)." *SE*, Vol. 12, 1958: 123–144.

_____. (1913b). "Zur Einleitung der Behandlung (Weitere Ratschläge zur Technik der Psychoanalyse I)." *Studienausgabe*: 181–203.

_____. (1914a). "Remembering, Repeating and Working-Through (Further Recommendations on the Technique of Psycho-Analysis II)." *SE*, Vol. 12, 1958: 147–156.

_____. (1914b). "Erinnern, Wiederholen, und Durcharbeiten (Weitere Ratschläge zur Technik der Psychoanalyse II)." *Studienausgabe*: 205–215.

_____. (1915a). "Observations on Transference-Love (Further Recommendations on the Technique of Psycho-Analysis III)." *SE*, Vol. 12, 1958: 159–171.

_____. (1915b). "Bemerkungen über die Übertragungsliebe (Weitere Ratschläge zur Technik der Psychoanalyse III)." *Studienausgabe*: 217–230.

_____. (1916–1917). *Introductory Lectures on Psycho-Analysis*. *SE*, Vols. 15 & 16, 1961.

_____. (1918). "From the History of an Infantile Neurosis." *SE*, Vol. 17, 1955: 7–122.

_____. (1919a). "Lines of Advance in Psycho-Analytic Therapy." *SE*, Vol. 17, 1955: 159–168.

_____. (1919b). "Wege der psychoanalytischen Therapie." *Studienausgabe*: 239–249.

_____. (1925). *An Autobiographical Study*. *SE*, Vol. 20, 1959: 1–74.

_____. (1926a). "The Question of Lay Analysis." *SE*, Vol. 20, 1959: 183–258.

_____. (1926b). "Die Frage der Laienanalyse." *Studienausgabe*: 271–341.

_____. (1937a). "Analysis Terminable and Interminable." *SE*, Vol. 23, 1964: 209–253.

_____. (1937b). "Die endliche und die unendliche Analyse." *Studienausgabe*: 351–392.

_____ . (1937c). "Constructions in Analysis." *SE*, Vol. 23, 1964: 255–269.

_____ . (1937d). "Konstruktionen in der Analyse." *Studienausgabe*: 393–406.

_____ . (1940a). *An Outline of Psycho-Analysis*. *SE*, Vol. 23, 1964: 139–207.

_____ . (1940b). "Die psychoanalytische Technik." Aus: *Abriss der Psychoanalyse. Studienausgabe*: 407–421.

Gardiner, M. (Ed.). (1971). *The Wolf-Man*. New York: Basic Books.

Gay, P. (1988). *Freud: A Life for Our Time*. New York: Norton.

Gedo, J. E., & Goldberg, A. (1973). *Models of the Mind*. Chicago and London: University of Chicago Press.

Gill, M. (1982). *Analysis of Transference* (Vol 1). New York: International Universities Press.

Glenn, J. (1980). "Freud's Adolescent Patients: Katharina, Dora, and the 'Homosexual Woman.'" In M. Kanzer & J. Glenn (Eds.), *Freud and His Patients*. New York: Aronson.

Goetz, B. (1975). "That Is All I Have to Say About Freud: Bruno Goetz's Reminiscences of Sigmund Freud." *International Review of Psycho-Analysis*, 2: 139–143.

Gray, P. (1994). *The Ego and Analysis of Defense*. Northvale, NJ: Aronson.

Greenson, R. (1967). *The Technique and Practice of Psychoanalysis* (Vol. 1). New York: International Universities Press.

Grinker, R. (1940). "Reminiscences of a Personal Contact with Freud." *American Journal of Orthopsychiatry*, 10: 850–855.

Hartmann, H. (1951). "Technical Implications of Ego Psychology." *Psychoanalytic Quarterly*, 20: 31–43.

Haynal, A. (1989). *Controversies in Psychoanalytic Method*. New York: New York University Press.

Holland, N. (1969). "Freud and H.D." *International Journal of Psycho-Analysis*, 50(3): 309–315.

Hughes, H. S. (1975). *The Sea Change*. New York: Harper & Row.

Jacoby, R. (1983). *The Repression of Psychoanalysis: Otto Fenichel and the Political Freudians*. New York: Basic Books.

Jones, E. (1953). *The Life and Work of Sigmund Freud: The Formative Years and the Great Discoveries, 1856–1900* (Vol. 1). New York: Basic Books.

_____ . (1955). *The Life and Work of Sigmund Freud: Years of Maturity, 1901–1919* (Vol. 2). New York: Basic Books.

_____ . (1957). *The Life and Work of Sigmund Freud: The Last Phase, 1919–1939* (Vol. 3). New York: Basic Books.

_____ . (Ed.). (1959). *Sigmund Freud: Collected Papers* (Vols. I–V). New York: Basic Books.

Kanzer, M. (1952). "The Transference Neurosis of the Rat Man." *Psychoanalytic Quarterly*, 21: 181–189.

_____ . (1979). "Development in Psychoanalytic Technique." *Journal of the American Psychoanalytic Association*, 27: 327–374.

_____ . (1980). "Freud's 'Human Influence' on the Rat Man." In M. Kanzer & J. Glenn (Eds.), *Freud and His Patients*. New York: Aronson.

_____ , & Blum, H. P. (1967). "Classical Psychoanalysis since 1931." In B. B. Wolman (Ed.), *Psychoanalytic Techniques: A Handbook for the Practicing Psychoanalyst*. New York: Basic Books.

Kardiner, A. (1945). *The Psychological Frontiers of Society*. New York: Columbia University Press.

———. (1977). *My Analysis with Freud: Reminiscences*. New York: Norton.

Khan, M. (1973). "Mrs. Alix Strachey: An Obituary." *International Journal of Psycho-Analysis, 54*: 370.

Kris, E. (1951). "Ego Psychology and Interpretation in Psychoanalytic Therapy." *Psychoanalytic Quarterly, 20*: 15–30.

Lampl-de Groot, J. (1976). "Personal Experiences with Psychoanalytic Technique and Theory During the Last Half Century." *Psychoanalytic Study of the Child, 31*: 283–296.

Langs, R. (1980). "The Misalliance Dimension in the Case of the Rat Man." In M. Kanzer & J. Glenn (Eds.), *Freud and His Patients*. New York: Aronson.

Laplanche, J., & Pontalis, J.-B. (1967). *The Language of Psycho-Analysis*. (D. Nicholson-Smith, Trans.). New York: Norton, 1973.

Lichtenberg, J., & Galler, F. (1987). "The Fundamental Rule: A Study of Current Usage." *Journal of the American Psychoanalytic Association, 35*: 47–76.

Lipton, S. D. (1977). "The Advantages of Freud's Technique As Shown in His Analysis of the Rat Man." *International Journal of Psycho-Analysis, 58*: 255–274.

Lohser, B. (1988). *Freud's Psychoanalytic Technique: A Re-Evaluation*. Unpublished doctoral dissertation, The Wright Institute, Berkeley, CA.

Masson, J. (Ed. and Trans.). (1985). *The Complete Letters of Sigmund Freud to Wilhelm Fliess, 1887–1904*. Cambridge, MA: Harvard University Press.

Miller, E. J., & Rice, A. K. (1967). *Systems of Organization*. London: Tavistock.

Mitscherlich, A., Richards, A., & Strachey, J. (Eds.). (1982). "Editorische Einleitung zu den behandlungstechnischen Schriften von 1911 bis 1915 [1914]." In *Sigmund Freud: Schriften zur Behandlungstechnik. Studienausgabe* (Ergänzungsband). Frankfurt am Rhein: Fischer.

Momigliano, L. (1987). "A Spell in Vienna: But Was Freud a Freudian? An Investigation into Freud's Technique Between 1920 and 1938, Based on the Published Testimony of Former Analysands." *International Review of Psycho-Analysis, 14*: 373–389.

Money-Kyrle, R. E. (1979). "Looking Backwards and Forwards." *International Review of Psychoanalysis, 6*: 265–271.

Nacht, S. (1958). "Variations in Technique. Panel Discussion." *International Journal of Psycho-Analysis, 39*: 235–237.

Newton, P. M. (1971). "Abstinence as a Role Requirement in Psychotherapy." *Psychiatry: Journal for the Study of Interpersonal Processes, 34*(4): 391–400.

———. (1973a). "Social Structure and Process in Psychotherapy: A Sociopsychological Approach to Transference, Resistance and Change." *International Journal of Psychiatry, 2*: 480–512.

———. (1973b). "Author's Reply." *International Journal of Psychiatry, 11*: 523–526.

———. (1989). "Free Association and the Division of Labor in Psychoanalytic Treatment," *Psychoanalytic Psychology, 6*: 31–46.

———. (1992a). "A Social System Approach to the Psychoanalytic Treatment of Personality Disorders." *Psychiatry: Interpersonal and Biological Processes, 55*: 66–78.

_____. (1992b). "Freud's Mid-Life Crisis." *Psychoanalytic Psychology*, 9: 447–475.

_____. (1995). *Freud: From Youthful Dream to Mid-Life Crisis*. New York: Guilford Press.

_____, & Levinson, D. J. (1973). "The Work Group Within the Organization: A Socio-Psychological Approach." *Psychiatry*, 36, 87–114.

Orgel, S. (1995). "A Classic Revisited: K. R. Eissler's 'The Effect of the Structure of the Ego on Psychoanalytic Technique.' " *Psychoanalytic Quarterly*, 64: 551–567.

Ornston, D. (Ed.). (1992). *Translating Freud*. New Haven, CT: Yale University Press.

Pulver, S. (1974). "Freud and Third-Party Payment: A Historical Note." *American Journal of Psychiatry*, 131(12): 1400–1402.

Racker, H. (1968). *Transference and Countertransference*. New York: International Universities Press.

Rangell, L. (1974). "A Psychoanalytic Perspective Leading Currently to the Compromise of Integrity." *International Journal of Psycho-Analysis*, 55: 3–12.

Rice, A. K. (1963). *The Enterprise and Its Environment*. London: Tavistock.

Riviere, J. (1939). "An Intimate Impression." In H. M. Ruitenbeek (Ed.), *Freud As We Knew Him*. Detroit: Wayne State University Press, 1973.

_____. (1956). "A Character Trait of Freud's." In H. M. Ruitenbeek (Ed.), *Freud As We Knew Him*. Detroit: Wayne State University Press, 1973.

Roazen, P. (1975). *Freud and His Followers*. New York: Knopf.

Ruitenbeek, H. M. (Ed.). (1973). *Freud As We Knew Him*. Detroit: Wayne State University Press.

Schröter, M. (Ed.). (1986). *Sigmund Freud: Briefe an Wilhelm Fliess, 1887–1904*. Frankfurt am Rhein: Fischer.

Stern, A. (1922). "Some Personal Psychoanalytic Experiences with Professor Freud." *New York State Journal of Medicine*, 22(1): 21–25.

Stone, L. (1961). *The Psychoanalytic Situation: An Examination of Its Development and Essential Nature*. New York: International Universities Press.

Strachey, J. (1934). "The Nature of the Therapeutic Action of Psycho-Analysis." *International Journal of Psycho-Analysis*, 15: 127–159.

Thompson, G. (1994). *The Truth About Freud's Technique: The Encounter with the Real*. New York: University Press.

Valenstein, A. (1979). "The Concept of 'Classical' Psychoanalysis." *Journal of the American Psychoanalytic Association*, 27: 113–136.

Voth, H. (1972). "Some Effects of Freud's Personality on Psycho-Analytic Theory and Technique." *International Journal of Psychiatry*, 10(4): 48–61.

Wallerstein, R. (1995). *The Talking Cures*. New Haven, CT: Yale University Press.

Weiss, S. (1980). "Reflections and Speculations on the Psychoanalysis of the Rat Man." In M. Kanzer & J. Glenn (Eds.), *Freud and His Patients*. New York: Aronson.

Wortis, J. (1954). *Fragments of an Analysis with Freud*. New York: Aronson, 1984.

Zetzel, E. (1966). "1965: Additional Notes upon a Case of Obsessional Neurosis: Freud 1909." *International Journal of Psycho-Analysis*, 47: 123–129.

Index